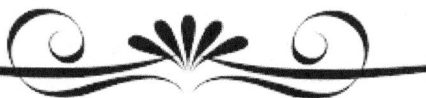

I0102476

This essay makes the claim that the controlling theater of human evolution has been the emotions and motivations that comprise the mind. I first illustrate how a handful of ancient emotions and motivations break down into the symptoms of major mental illnesses. I then assemble these "emotional fossils" into an evolutionary narrative of the human *mind*.

Six million years ago, amid deteriorating climates threatening extinction, the target of natural selection decisively shifted from the *fittest* ape individuals to the *most productive associations among* human individuals. From the very beginning, the coordination of divided labor has been the crucial human adaptation. To permit the intimate engagement required for this teamwork to emerge and thrive, collective instincts for justice were evolved and refined.

Then 300,000 years ago, our own species evolved an intense motivation to be admired by—and to admire—one another. The self-sustaining evolution of this two-way force of attraction has relentlessly drawn us into increasingly larger intercommunicating populations igniting the maintenance and natural selection of know-how across generations.

This 130-page essay provides an intuitive understanding, not just of the known science of mental illness and human evolution, but also of the motivations underlying our capacities for self-awareness and complex language. An optimistic and progressive vision of human nature emerges as deeply rooted in the legacy of justice from our ancestral species.

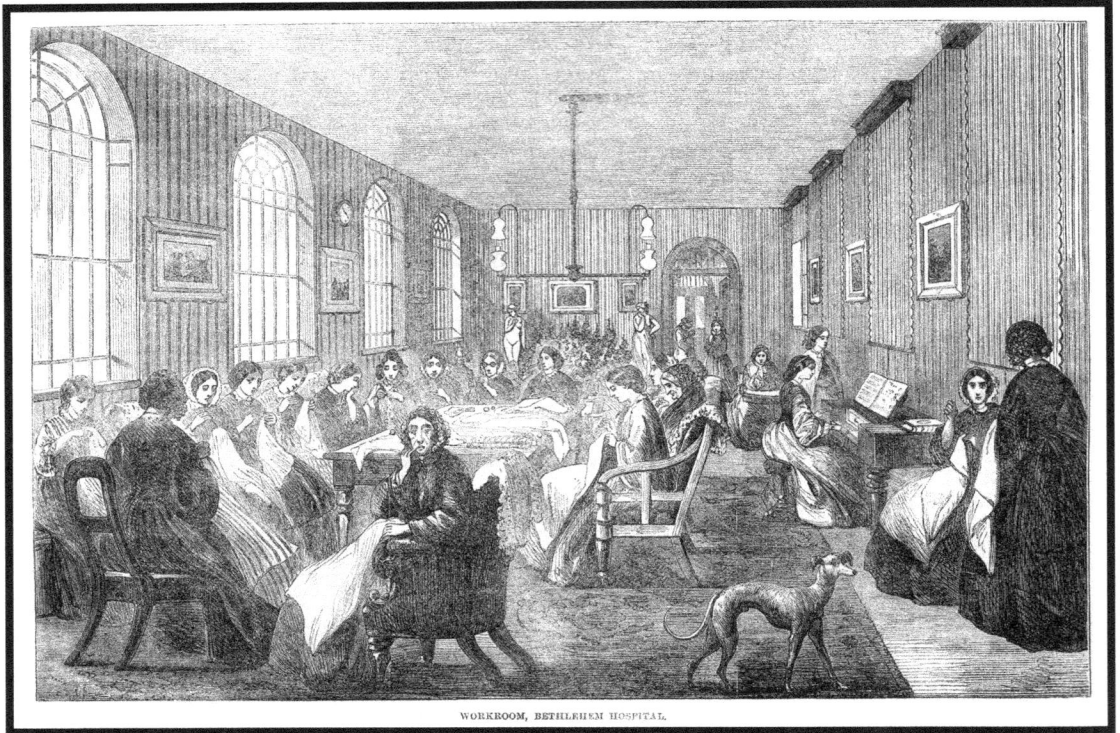

WORKROOM, BETHLEHEM HOSPITAL.

WORKROOM (1860)
Bethlem Royal Hospital of London
First psychiatric hospital founded 1330

...you find yourself in a long and wide gallery, on either side of which are a large number of little cells where lunatics of every description are shut up, and you can get a sight of these poor creatures, little windows being let into the doors. On holidays numerous persons of both sexes, but belonging generally to the lower classes, visit this hospital and amuse themselves watching these unfortunate wretches, who often give them cause for laughter.

—Account of Bethlem during 1725 tour of London's sights

EMOTIONAL FOSSILS

MENTAL ILLNESS AND HUMAN EVOLUTION

JOHN V WYLIE, MD

WHY WE BECAME
HUMAN

Olney, Maryland

To Richard

"Inside everyone is the same."
—*Dalai Lama*

CONTENTS

PART ONE
EMOTIONAL FOSSILS

PART TWO
MIND MEETS MATTER

PART THREE
DESTINY'S CHILDREN

EMOTIONAL FOSSILS

INTRODUCTION

The miracle of our capacities to think has been woven through the millennia upon the evolving loom of how we feel. This book—really an essay—is a sustained argument for the proposition that the *subjective experience* of major mental illnesses contains valid empirical evidence that, from the very first stirrings of becoming human some 50 million years ago, our unique intelligence has evolved in response to environments comprised solely of emotions and motivations.

Although the essay is not about the treatment of mental illness, please keep in mind its medical mission in the background. The clinical goal of the essay is to diagnose and treat the insult of social stigma that has always been part of the suffering of mental illnesses. My aim is to humanize these conditions by revealing that they are disorders of the very emotions and motivations that have rendered us human throughout the epic struggle of our evolutionary journey. Once the intimate connection between mental illness and all that is human in us becomes clear, so will the sentiment that those among us living with these terrible afflictions should be respected for paying a price—not just for our humanity, but for our ascendant mind with which we have been so richly endowed.

It is not generally understood that there is virtually no direct scientific knowledge about how the mind of apes evolved into the human mind. Huge amounts of scientific knowledge about the minds of apes and the minds of humans (particularly children) are neatly being stacked upon the cliffs on either side of the six-million-year canyon of time that separates apes from us. But it is within this vast silent chasm that all human ancestors, whose ghosts animate the very core of us, forged our destiny.

Michael Tomasello, perhaps the foremost scientist on mind evolution, states,

The main problem is that collaboration, communication, and thinking do not fossilize, so we will always be in a position of speculation about such behavioral phenomena, as well as the specific events that were critical to their evolution. Most critical, we do not know how much contemporary great apes have changed from their common ancestor with humans because there are basically no relevant fossils from this era (*A Natural History of Human Thinking*, 2014).

Similar to psychoanalysis, I have examined the subjective experience of the most severe psychiatric illnesses, but I have interpreted them in the context of our species' evolution instead of childhood development. The disruption of normal mental function in mental illness does not so much distort, but rather greatly magnifies emotions and motivations so elemental that they can be pieced together into a narrative of the inner experience of human evolution. Two forms of major depression reflect the rise of social fears in primates some 50 million years ago, and schizophrenia disables the collective system of communication likely to have appeared with our ancestral species. The manic phase of bipolar disorder is linked by pathology in cognitively demanding speech to motivations that distinguish our own species. The essay humanizes the scientized fields of psychiatry and human evolution by relating them to emotions and motivations we all know intimately.

Narrative truth

"What brings you in today?" you ask after a new patient sits down in your office. The first order of business is a chronology of the present illness. Precisely when did the problem start? What was happening at that moment and more generally in his/her life at that time? Then the present illness is placed into the wider narrative of the person's life history. As the person talks, you attempt to causally link the sequence of events into a narrative with several possible diagnoses. To me, this fascinating exercise never gets old.

In his book, *The Why of Things*: *Causality in Science, Medicine, and Life* (2013), Johns Hopkins psychiatrist Peter Rabins states, "Causal narratives seek to knit together disparate observations, facts, and events into a coherent and inclusive whole that convincingly links later events to prior events." Rabins calls this *narrative truth*. In other fields of medicine, after arriving at several possible diagnostic narratives, the empirical certainty of the scientific method is martialed by obtaining lab tests to settle on a single diagnosis. However, the value of a given test is called into question if the results are not consistent with the history; perhaps the wrong test was administered.

The task of this essay is akin to the process employed by Freud in constructing his psychoanalytic system. Freud's task was to reconstruct the symptoms he observed in his patients into a causal narrative of childhood development. My task in this essay is to employ the symptoms I observed to indicate a causal narrative in our species' deep evolution. This method is not a mere technique. Rabins cites evidence that the ability to construct and recognize causal narratives has been physically evolved into our brains:

> For me, though, the most convincing evidence that the distinction [of the narrative method] has value and *says something about the structure of knowledge* [my italics] is the fact that the narrative approach is present in all cultures and used by all individuals, whereas the methods of science are a relatively recent invention.

> Studies carried out by the neuroscientists Roger Sperry and Michael Gazzaniga offer further support for this view. They examined patients who had previously undergone "split brain" surgery—that is, had the large fiber bundle that connects the two hemispheres of their brain severed in an attempt to stop the spread of seizure discharges from one side to the other—and they found evidence that there is a "center" in the brain, near or overlapping the language area in the left hemisphere, that "makes" connections between disparate pieces of evidence. This strongly suggests that the human brain is constructed to carry out narrative reasoning and that the linking of facts into a narrative causal web is innate (p. 167).

Stigma and the fear of contagion

In my first year of medical school, the tropical disease professor had the entire class, one by one, touch the hands of a woman with Henson's disease before telling us that the common name is leprosy.

Biblical leprosy is the prototype of stigma. *The Land and the Book* was published in 1859 and was only outsold by *Uncle Tom's Cabin*. Written by Rev. William McClure Thompson, it related his experiences as an American missionary to the Holy Land. Note that the analogy of leprosy to sin is driven by the fear of contagion.

> . . . There are many most striking analogies between [leprosy] and that more deadly leprosy of sin which has involved our whole race in one common

ruin. It is feared as contagious; it is certainly and inevitably hereditary; it is loathsome and polluting; its victim is shunned by all as unclean; it is most deceitful in its action. Who can fail to find in all this a most affecting type of man's moral leprosy? (Vol 2: 519).

The tranquility of care depicted in the *Workroom* shown on the frontispiece of this essay is contrasted with the degradation portrayed in the comments below about the legendary Bethlem Hospital as a sight-not-to-be missed when traveling to 18th century London. The amusement commented upon in the description introduces the stigma of mental illness. It is tempting to compare the entertainment of those onlookers to a circus sideshow, but those circus attractions are mere physical abnormalities that counter any sense of personal identity with them.

In stark contrast, the jarring dissonance of mental illness strikes alarming chords deep inside core feelings that trigger the dread of contagion, which is at the heart of stigma. It is possible that the fear of contagion has been naturally selected for the benefits of avoiding infectious diseases. The abiding reaction of stigma seeks to quarantine the carriers of these diseases far beyond physical sequestration—to bar them from our empathy as well. This essay reveals that our disturbing inner resonance with mental illness in actuality springs from a deep kinship, which, when understood, can naturally be embraced and even honored.

The word *crazy* arose as a stigmatic reference to the mentally ill in the early 1600s and proceeded to metastasize into general use as a pejorative term, having recently inherited the misogynistic baggage of the now-banned *hysterical*. The jazz age cooled the slur down with *crazy rhythm*, recently branching into the unambiguously positive *crazy good*. This follows the romantic, Dionysian (lunar) strand of attitudes toward the mentally ill—a complete fiction—coupled with the idea that *madness* is next to genius (some truth there). *Nut job* and *whacko* are the young punks on the block, but *psycho* has muscled its way into being the alpha denigration[1] of the mentally ill, and then the follow-up, "They ought to lock him/her up!"

In examining the word *crazy* as a proxy for the vicissitudes of stigma, the fear of dangerous fanaticism (crazy radicals) is specifically associated with schizophre-

---

[1] Latin dēnigrātus is the past participle of dēnigrāre, *to blacken*.

nia's hallmark of delusions (false beliefs), which occasionally do motivate violence. This association is not ignored and will be placed in the perspective of the normal human function that breaks down in schizophrenia.

As we learned with the AIDS epidemic, the most effective treatment for the stigma of an illness is effective treatment for the illness itself. However, effective treatment follows from an understanding of the biological mechanisms of the disease. Unfortunately, as I will illustrate, a physiological or genetic understanding of mental illness is not yet in sight.

Darwin

Well do I remember my excitement in the spring of 1988 when, after over a decade of thinking in complete isolation about the relevance of Darwin to psychiatry, I happened upon an article by psychiatrist Randolph Nesse at the University of Michigan titled "The evolutionary functions of repression and the ego defenses." After contacting him, Nesse cordially invited me to attend a meeting he organized in Ann Arbor that launched the Human Behavior and Evolution Society, which continues rigorously to peer review multidisciplinary scientific papers for their journal. Now to cap off a remarkable career, Nesse has published *Good Reasons for Bad Feelings, Insights from the Frontier of Evolutionary Psychiatry* (2019), a fascinating and fun-to-read compendium of thirty years of science on psychiatric disorders and existential angst from an evolutionary perspective. This essay is meant to further the general project of engaging medicine more robustly into the Darwinian paradigm that has so revolutionized the rest of biology.

Darwin initiated the evolutionary study of emotions in *The Expression of the Emotions in Man and Animals* (1872). This is the last paragraph of this final treatise:

> We have also seen that expression in itself, or the language of the emotions, as it has sometimes been called, is certainly of importance for the welfare of mankind. To understand, as far as possible, the source or origin of the various expressions which may be hourly seen on the faces of the men around us, not to mention the domesticated animals, ought to possess much interest for us.

Nesse claims that Darwin's book, ". . . emphasized communication [expression] but neglected physiological, cognitive, and motivational functions. In short, Darwin's book about emotions really is anti-Darwinian." Nesse seeks to understand the strategic benefits to the *individual*[2] of a given emotion, whereas I am focused on the mystery of why and how humans have evolved to *express* all their emotions.

Paul Ekman has devoted his career to the study of facial expression (2007, 2013). He confirms the importance Darwin assigns to "expression in itself" in human emotion: "It is part of our evolutionary heritage that we signal [express] when each emotion begins." Although modern humans vary in their capacity to express their emotions, and emotional expressions differ between cultures (Crivelli et al., 2016), the universal default expectation of others is that their expressed emotions are transparent (Levine, 2014). In Chapter 8, I will present evidence from studies of developing children that human language was naturally selected for benefits of collaborative foraging.

I propose that human evolution is marked by a decisive shift in natural selection's target from fitness of individuals to productivity of relationships among individuals in which the language of expressed emotions plays the central role. Human emotions changed from promoting individual fitness to coordinating productive teamwork among individuals, which I argue is the central human adaptation.

This essay, like Freudian psychoanalysis, examines and analyzes the *quality* of *subjective experience* in emotions. The most difficult dimension to grasp in this essay is the shift in the evolutionary arena from physical environments to social environments—from behaviors and cognitions ("mental behaviors") to emotions and motivations. Based on the psychoanalysis of five mental illnesses, this essay proposes the evolution of all our ancestral human species was predominantly influenced by a social environment comprised of collective emotions and motivations. This general proposal provides a far simpler and more coherent explanation for the principal facts of paleoanthropology (Chapter 8) and our unique mental capacities (Chapter 10), than does the classical perspective of individual-level evolution in response to physical environments.

---

[2] Or, as will be explained, benefits to genes that blood relatives have in common, called *kin selection.*

I propose that two major forms of depression reveal the collective emotions that have bound social groups together since the very dawn of primate sociality: the fear of interpersonal *separation* and the fear of *entrapment at the bottom or periphery of groups*. Central to this theory is my proposal that schizophrenia disables the communication of collective norms from groups, a function so highly developed and fundamental to modern social organization that it must have been present in the ancient, perhaps the most ancient, ancestral species of our tribe Hominini.[4] Similarly, the manic phase of bipolar disorder reveals emotions and motivations central to the evolution of our own *Homo sapiens* species.

Melding these insights with the science and theory of evolution, it is clear there were two reconfigurations in the dynamics of social emotion resulting in two evolutionary transitions in social structure: one from apes to hominins about six million years ago, and the other denoting the appearance of our own species three hundred thousand years ago.

The salutary impact on the blight of stigma lies in Chapters 8 and 10. The same experiences of mental illness stigmatized through the ages become ancient beacons illuminating a fresh and uplifting vision of *who we are*. Apart from hopes for more effective treatments, in my dreams I go to a time when the profound humanness of mental illness is felt and also honored.

---

[4] Our traditional biological classification as a *hominid family* (family Hominidae) was recently changed to a *hominin tribe*.

PART ONE

EMOTIONAL FOSSILS

Note to the reader. Before I proceed into clinical material, I need to explain a professional convention used in this essay which might be interpreted as dehumanizing: the practice of calling everyone under medical care a "patient." I ask you to understand that I am writing this essay as a physician. When I use "patient," I refer to the covenant of trust that is the doctor-patient relationship, within the sanctuary of which the inner experiences of mental illness were disclosed to me. The word, patient is derived from Latin meaning "one who suffers." With respect to this root meaning, it is beneficial to refer to (and think of) those with chronic mental illness as living with and dealing with their medical condition, rather than as (passive) sufferers, similar to attitudes toward anyone coping with a chronic medical condition.

CHAPTER 1

RELATIONSHIP TO BRAIN SCIENCE

Chemical imbalance and all in the genes?

The neurochemistry of mental illness has revealed a jungle of complexity with major problems discriminating among cause, compensation, and effect, and virtually all our knowledge stems from the effects of drugs. As Thomas R. Insel, the former director of the U.S. National Institute of Mental Health (NIMH), said in *Science,*

> We just don't know enough. Research and development in this area has been almost entirely dependent on the serendipitous discoveries of medications. From the get-go, none of it was ever based on an understanding of any of the illnesses involved (Miller, 2012).

The genetics of mental illness, and particularly schizophrenia, are fraught with the history of the eugenics movement of the 1920s and '30s. In 1928, twenty states had compulsory sterilization laws, most including "lunatics"[5] among the target population. This sterilization movement was based on the assumption that mental illness is caused by a small number of recessive Mendelian genes. The fallaciousness of this idea became clear in Hitler's ghastly effort to eliminate schizophrenia in Germany:

> It is estimated that between 220,000 and 269,500 individuals with schizophrenia were sterilized or killed. This total represents between 73% and 100% of all individuals with schizophrenia living in Germany between 1939 and 1945. Postwar studies of the prevalence of schizophrenia in Germany reported low rates, as expected. However, postwar rates of the incidence [new cases] of schizophrenia in Germany were unexpectedly high (Torrey and Yolken, 2010).

---

[5] The term "lunatic," as in "loony bin," has roots in archaic, stigmatic notions that mental illness is related to lunar cycles.

Franz Josef Kallmann, an advocate of compulsory sterilization in Germany, fled to the U.S. in 1936 where he later conducted seminal twin studies. He found that the incidence of schizophrenia rose from about 1% in the general population to an 86% co-morbidity in identical twins (Kallmann, 1946). This is in the same range as a large recent study placing the genetically inherited component at 79% (Hilker, 2017). It is now acknowledged that, like most other complex illnesses, mental illness is caused by many genes of small effect, and combinations of risk factors in each family lineage might be virtually unique.

Partially as a result of difficulties isolating causes within the flux of brain chemistry, there has been a recent effort to decipher the presumably more stable genetics of mental illness. Published in *Science* by The BrainSTORM Consortium (2018) at the Center for Brain Science at Harvard University, a study conducted by hundreds of investigators over five years and involving more than one million genomes provided telling results. Whereas the neurological conditions demonstrated distinctive unshared risks for each disorder in their genetic underpinnings, the genetic risk for psychiatric disorders could not be distinguished from one another. As a group, it correlated only with the personality category of neuroticism[6] and with developmental cognitive deficits (possibly secondary to the neuroticism). This essentially negative finding led to the following conclusion:

> The high degree of genetic correlation among the psychiatric disorders adds further evidence that current clinical diagnostics do not reflect specific genetic etiology for these disorders and that genetic risk factors for psychiatric disorders do not respect clinical diagnostic boundaries. Rather, this finding suggests a more interconnected genetic etiology [from neuroticism], in contrast to that of neurologic disorders, and underscores the need to refine psychiatric diagnostics.

Clearly this study, in which the genetics of mental illnesses are indistinguishable from each other, does not provide a path to refine psychiatric diagnostics to fit underlying genetic causes.

---

[6] Neuroticism is one of the "Big Five" personality traits. Individuals who score high on neuroticism are more likely to be anxious, self-pitying, tense, touchy, unstable, worrying, with fluctuating moods (McCrae and John, 1992).

Meanwhile the even more ambitious ongoing PsychENCODE project, organized by the National Institutes of Health in 2015, attempts to unravel differences among psychiatric illnesses in the non-coding regulatory and epigenetic portions of the genome. The first set of papers published as the cover story in the December 14, 2018, issue of *Science* provides an enormous data set demonstrating how the expression of disparate genes with common functions congregate in genome "modules." Although most (but not all) psychiatric geneticists accept that this research is moving in the right direction, there is general agreement that the path to a genetically mediated mechanism for mental illness is not yet understood.

Functional disorders

It is easy to forget that all this high-powered research is performed on illnesses that are almost completely defined by patients reporting their experience of the symptoms. So far, these studies are entirely consistent with the *functional* model of mental illness in which the primary pathology does not lie in genetic mutations but is considered a malfunction at the highest level of brain integration, the psychological level. This was the predominant view during most of the 20th century, including the early years of my practice in the 1970s.

My functional proposal is that the variation in the symptoms of different mental illnesses are not determined by the pathology, which is the same for all, but by the normal segment of emotional function from which each illness is derived. In an editorial titled "Genomics Is Not Enough" in *Science* (2011), Aravinda Chakravarti, a professor at the McKusick-Nathans Institute of Genetic Medicine at Johns Hopkins University, offers two possibilities for the genetics of a given illness:

> Each individual is genomically unique, with DNA variation in our genomes serving as markers of our ancestries. Are each individual's biology and disease also unique? Or does sequence diversity in any disease coalesce into a smaller set of common functional deficiencies?

I propose that the genetics underlying the emotional functions that break down into each mental illness, including risk factors for their common pathology, are unique to each family lineage.[7]

As mentioned, the primary human adaptation from the very beginning has been the decisive advantage of communal (as opposed to individual) function evolved in response to the *ecology* of highly evolved social environments comprised of collective emotions and motivations. In Chapter 7, I will discuss how natural selection for collective functioning has involved predominantly the maintenance within individuals of optimal *balances* between spectra of competing temperaments (e.g., aggression and fearfulness) over long periods of time. This rebalancing process not only serves to sustain and refine emotional modulation,[8] but also to generate the diversity of temperaments required for the productive benefits of divided labor. This centrally human evolutionary process of rebalancing, generation after generation, is uniquely achieved in each family lineage by remixing existing constellations of genes controlling temperament. Because risk factors for mental illness involve imbalances in temperament (neuroticism), they too are unique to family lineages.

Evolutionary psychoanalysis

I use the term phenomenology to refer simply to the study of our inner experiences. The greatest 20th-century psychiatrists were phenomenologists. Their basic "data" were descriptions by patients of their subjective experiences of these illnesses. Of course, the genius who spawned the phenomenological view that dominated psychiatry for most of the 20th century and led to psychoanalytic theory was Sigmund Freud. I ask my psychoanalytic colleagues to consider evolutionary psychoanalysis to be a sister phenomenological system of knowledge similarly obtained by the empathetic method but applied to the larger context of human evolution.

---

[7] This is consistent with the high concordance rate in identical twins and the heritability of mental illnesses in general.

[8] The *timbre* (tonal quality) *of* seriousness is a modulated balance of emotion.

Whereas Freudian psychoanalysis rests on the assumption that childhood development is the cause of the mature id/superego dynamic (and its ailments), evolutionary psychoanalysis views these same developmental stages as the result of millions of years of evolution in accordance with the principles of natural selection (and others) established by Charles Darwin. This essay does not contradict existing psychoanalytic theory,[9] but it has a completely different focus because of its evolutionary approach.

The foundation of the Freudian psychoanalytic system is the self-evidence of Freud's fundamental vision of the division of the mind into the conscious (small) realm and the unconscious (large) realm and the central dynamic between id (sex and aggression) and superego (guilt and shame). The authority of this theory is established democratically by a critical mass of key individuals deciding whether the descriptions of the functioning of our emotions and motivations resonate and ring true. Both Freudian psychoanalysis and the system explained in this essay rely on information that is transmitted and verified by the highly evolved human capacity for empathy. I will demonstrate that the basis for empathy lies in the evolution of the collective mentality that defines our humanity. As the Dalai Lama states in the quotation at the beginning of this essay, "Inside everyone is the same."

For thirty-five years, I examined the inner experience of the major mental illnesses through the lens of evolution. I concluded that each of these conditions is derived from a discrete bundle of normal emotional function that has escaped from its usual regulated role into a sustained state of pathological hyperactivity, which then dominates and disables the totality of mental function.

---

[9] An exception is that I offer an alternative definition of *ego* in Chapter 9.

CHAPTER 2

FEEDBACK REVERBERATION

The empathetic method

The effect on my practice of my interest in evolutionary psychoanalysis was a scrupulous attention to patients' descriptions of how they experienced their illnesses. I was constantly deepening a composite essence of the experience of each illness. I never considered this activity a treatment and refrained from delving into these ideas with patients. However, I sought to ease these people's fear about their alien experiences by communicating that they were well known to me. In addition, my interest engendered my gratitude for being granted frank access to their inner life.

Diagnosing mental illness has always been an attempt to discriminate empathetically symptoms common to an illness. The experienced practitioner can gauge the quality of the emotional "harmonic" characteristic of each illness with more precision than the words that describe it. Here I explore the deep human meaning imbedded within the subjective experience of each mental disorder.

The objective of the empathetic examinations presented here is to provide detailed information about the specific segment of the normal emotional-and-motivational function from which each illness is derived. Five mental illnesses[10] provide insight into corresponding segments of normal function and how they fit together into an evolutionary narrative.

Pathological hyperactivity

In the genetic study cited above, neuroticism and cognitive deficits were found to be predispositions, or risk factors, for all major mental illnesses. Leaving aside the

---

[10] An evolutionary psychoanalysis of OCD, which has a clear relationship to function, has been omitted for the sake of brevity, and I do not have the requisite experience to evaluate autism.

cognitive deficits, neuroticism, or excessive moodiness, can be considered as a pan-dysregulation of emotions across the entire spectrum from fearfulness to aggression and everything in between. However, a large proportion of the population has "issues" controlling their moods and emotions under stressful circumstances for which they appropriately may seek therapy, including medications. Establishing a clear understanding of how to discriminate these *existential* difficulties from the pathological breakdown that characterizes all mental illness is a crucial step in understanding these illnesses.

The pathology of runaway feedback loops occurs when their regulation fails. The simplest examples of feedback regulation are hormonal systems in which a substance that stimulates the production of a hormone is inhibited by the hormone itself. As the level of the hormone becomes too high, it causes a decrease in the substance's level that stimulates the hormone's production, and thus the hormone's level is regulated downward.

Among the most common pathological mechanisms in medicine, such as at a molecular level in the regulation of cell growth in cancer, is the escape from this kind of feedback control into runaway, unregulated, positively reinforced feedback. I am proposing that this same pathological mechanism operates at the highest neuronal levels—the level at which emotions are experienced—in mental illness. In the following two chapters, I demonstrate how two forms of depression are the result of two normally functioning social fears devolving into unrestrained pathological feedback.

Consider two individuals arguing: each is making the other angrier, but each is also restrained by their fears of social repercussions; as the quarrel escalates, these restraints might fail and unfettered violence might ensue. The proclivity of some individuals to lash out into unrestrained aggression is at the heart of disorders of aggression, such as many that I encountered in my early practice in a prison environment. However, in depression it is the social fears which regulate aggressions that escalate into pathological hyperactivity.

What's in a name?

It is necessary to apply up front an official name that captures the essentials of the experiential pathology common to all mental illnesses. The analogy of a feedback loop between a microphone (input) and speaker (output) is appropriate because the element that escalates is sound, and the experience of emotions and motivations bear similarities to that of sound[11] in that both have inputs (emotion) and outputs (motivation). Although not a mental illness, the internal dynamics of stigmatizing individuals are comprised of the *input* of emotional contagion-dread from the mentally ill and the *output* of motivations to contain it. Mental illnesses occur when input and output escalate into a screeching pitch. This pathologically self-reinforcing mechanism is called *positive feedback*, but that term seems inappropriate for a process that causes the horror of mental illness, so I call it *feedback reverberation*.

The word "feedback" is well known in modern parlance and means an independent response from another party; for instance, we might say that we want to "bounce something off you." The word "reverberation" adds two elements to the concept of feedback. The first is forcefulness or intensity. The Latin root is the noun *verber*, which means a whip or lash; then the verb *verberare*, meaning to strike or beat, and *reverberare* means to strike back. The second element is that of a continuing push-back process, or vibration, regarding sound. The first entry in the *Oxford English Dictionary* is from Geoffrey Chaucer's *Summoner's Tale* (1604): "The rumbling of a fart and every soun Nys but of Eye reuerberacion." Translated: "The rumbling of a fart, and every sound, is nothing but the reverberation of air." And, as an earthy chord has been struck, another apt example of feedback reverberation is sex leading to orgasm. Much of mental illness can be compared to a sustained orgasm comprised of intensely painful fear. So in combining these two concepts, the interactive loop in feedback is further distinguished by rapidly escalating frequency and intensity of reverberation.

The *all-consuming* nature of the feedback reverberation experience is the crucial distinction between the mental illnesses discussed in this essay and either neuroticism or life's problems that lie in wait for us all. In the absence of mental illness, painful emotional experiences that are part of living a life can be alleviated by comprehending their meaning in the larger narrative in which the individual's past and present life is embedded. However, once the feedback reverberation process of mental illness sets in, all these moorings in the patient's life are ruptured and

---

[11] Accordingly, I sometimes refer to the increased "volume" of emotions in mental illness.

consumed by the screeching magnitude of suffering in the present moment—by feedback reverberation. In this sense, the word *crazy* can be used to stand for the radical degree to which pathological feedback reverberation is a break from normalcy. I am for limiting the use of *crazy* to this one sense, used with respect and without malice. I feel that limiting the meaning of a such a common word is more feasible than banning it.

The iconic image of *The Scream* (1893) by Edvard Munch accurately portrays the experience of major mental illness.

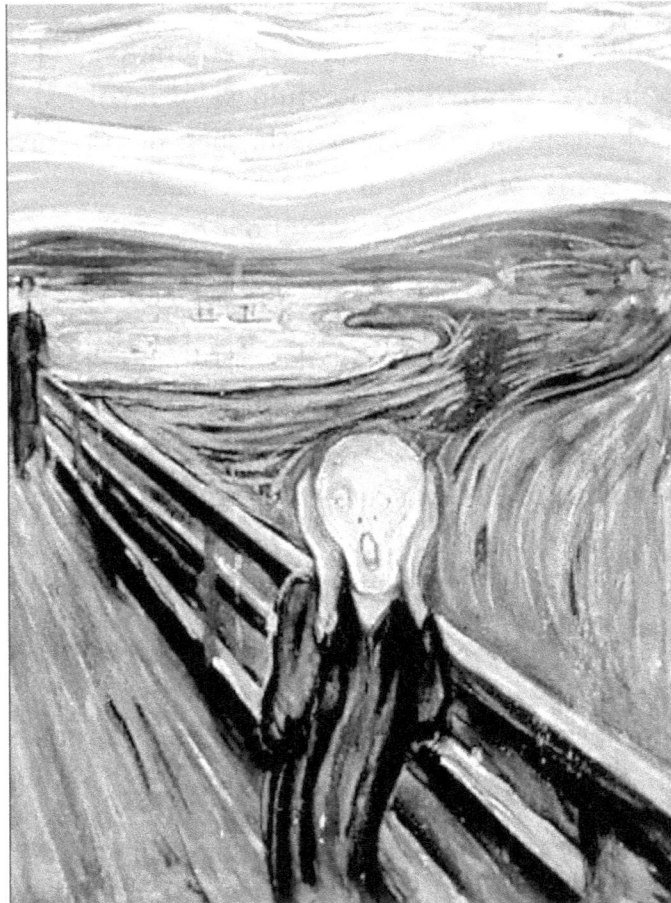

CHAPTER 3

SEPARATION

First things first

Midway through my career, apart from the "biological revolution," the psychoanalytic paradigm that mental illness is caused by emotions was partially supplanted by an alternative. A significant advance in "talking" psychotherapy was cognitive therapy pioneered by Aaron T. Beck (1967). Cognition pertains to intellectual activities involving thinking, reasoning, memory, and learning, as opposed to emotions and motivations. The premise behind cognitive therapy is disarmingly simple: it is not the patients' emotions that are disordered, but their belief systems and cognitive processes. The therapist attempts to enlist faculties of reason to convince patients that the emotionally laden cognitive beliefs they have (e.g., "I am stupid and worthless") are in fact false. The therapist points out various habitual cognitive errors produced by unconscious "automatic thinking."

Although Beck was a psychoanalytically trained psychiatrist, his treatment fit right in with the cognitive revolution going on in psychology and rapidly gained wide acceptance among clinical psychologists. Cognitive therapists principally target depression and anxiety disorders and have attracted well-deserved attention because they prove in controlled studies (to the degree that these studies can be controlled) that their treatment is at least as effective as drug treatment, and that combined treatment has the best outcomes. Here was an alternative paradigm to psychoanalytic theory as to how the mind (as opposed to the physiology of the brain) could break down into mental illness by means of cognitive dysfunction.

While I was so impressed by these studies I began referring many of my patients for co-treatment with cognitive therapists, after considering it, I rejected the idea that mental illnesses were caused by unconscious erroneous thinking. I could understand how entrenched cognitive assumptions about oneself over many years could distort one's self-image, but could not see how thoughts alone transform these false beliefs into the emotional intensity of mental illness. Countless times I witnessed patients suffering from melancholia, with convictions that their lives were irreparably ruined, improve with drug treatment, and simultaneously their cognitive attitudes about themselves almost invariably reverted to normal. It is clear to me that pathologically intense emotions distort cognitions in severe mental illnesses and not the other way around.

Just because a therapy is effective, it does not follow that whatever is being corrected by the therapy caused the illness in the first place. We have learned that lesson in psychiatry with psychiatric medications. We have a deep understanding of what and how neurotransmitter systems are altered by these medications, but we have also come to accept that this knowledge does not lead to an understanding of the causes of mental illnesses, which remain a mystery.

Atypical depression

I have before me the March 3, 1952, issue of *Life* magazine. On pages 20–21, there is a picture spread with the headline TB MILESTONE. The pictures are of a tuberculosis ward in Staten Island; one depicts a group of beds empty except for one occupied by a woman "who has difficulty walking." The next picture shows the patients, who were previously bedridden, laughing and dancing together in the corridor. Those patients had been placed on the drug iproniazid, which had been synthesized from leftover German V-2 benzene rocket fuel as an anti-tuberculosis medication. A psychiatrist noted the picture and correctly surmised that it was not the drug's beneficial effect on the TB bacillus that was producing the apparent mania in these patients, but a direct effect on the brain's emotional regulatory system. Iproniazid turned out to be toxic to the liver, but it led to the synthesis of the first two antidepressants, Parnate and Nardil, which are mono-amine oxidase inhibitors, or MAOIs.

Astonishingly, Parnate and Nardil remain the most powerful antidepressants available today. For example, Nardil was the only treatment that helped the writer David Foster Wallace, and rendered him virtually symptom-free for his most productive period. Artists often asked me whether psychiatric medication would impair their creativity. My answer was that perhaps it might, but not as much as mental illness does. Wallace stopped taking Nardil because he feared it was affecting his writing, but when he restarted, it was no longer effective. This unfortunate outcome is not unusual, and he ended up committing suicide. Writing was good therapy for Wallace, but in the end, it could not sustain him.

Early in their use, explosive increases in blood pressure in some patients were noted with these drugs, and they were temporarily removed from the market. They caused "hypertensive crises" by preventing the metabolism of tyramine, an amino acid found in aged foods, such as cheese. By the time Parnate and Nardil were placed back on the market with strict dietary restriction, the tricyclic antidepressants Tofranil and Elavil, developed from antihistamines, had been demonstrated to be effective in treating depression, but without the dangerous hypertensive problem. The MAOIs became (and continue to be) rarely used.

In the early 1960s, however, several psychiatric clinics in England continued using the MAOIs. Uniquely in the annals of medicine to my knowledge, these British psychiatrists defined an illness, a variety of depression, based on its specific therapeutic responsiveness to a drug, namely the MAOIs. They dubbed this condition atypical depression, in contrast to melancholic depression, or melancholia, which they suspected was a separate condition more treatable with the tricyclic antidepressants than MAOIs.

Ancient Greek physicians recognized melancholia as a disease. Any medical student should be able to recite its symptoms, including physical agitation and the so-called *vegetative* symptoms of insomnia, lack of interest in food, and weight loss. In addition, melancholic depression cannot be altered either by positive or negative circumstances or by events. Atypical depression as described by the British as responsive to MAOI medication, comprises anxiety, as opposed to physical agitation. The vegetative symptoms of melancholia are absent, and these patients often overeat and oversleep. Patients suffering from atypical depression are also reactive to ongoing interpersonal events, most notably to interpersonal rejection.

About the time that the English were defining atypical depression by its response to MAOIs, Donald Klein and his colleagues at Columbia University in New York initiated an interest in this same condition. They used the name *hysteroid dysphoria* to describe a syndrome that includes oversleeping and overeating in personalities with long-standing sensitivity to rejection. The Columbia group also emphasized that these patients, in contrast to those suffering from melancholic depression, were energized and brightened in response to positive interpersonal attention, even when depressed. In contrast to the emphasis on anxiety by the British, the Columbia group included fatigue as an important symptom in this kind of depression.

In 1988, the Columbia group published a major clinical research study showing that the MAOI Nardil is more effective than the tricyclic Tofranil in treating atypical depression. The distinction between the two types of depression became established. The diagnostic manual of The American Psychiatric Association in 1994 admitted atypical depression as a subtype of depression under its original English name.[12] To qualify as having atypical depression, the patient has to exhibit "mood reactivity (i.e., mood brightens in response to actual or potential positive events)" plus at least two of the following four symptoms: (1) overeating, (2) oversleeping, (3) "leaden paralysis (i.e., heavy, leaden feeling in arms or legs)," and (4) "long-standing pattern of interpersonal rejection sensitivity that results in social or occupational impairment."

Two symptoms attracted me to atypical depression. From its recognition as a clinical entity, it has been associated with rejection sensitivity. Typically, this kind of depression occurs after a patient has been rejected in a romantic relationship. Rejection sensitivity interested me because here was a temporary pathological emotional state caused by a permanent personality trait. Atypical depression was the initial example through which I came to understand that other mental illnesses were also manifestations of normal emotional traits, the regulation of which had failed, resulting in pathologically hyperactive emotional states. I reasoned that, because specific emotional traits could paralyze the patient's mental function when they broke down, these emotions played a key role not only in normal behavior but also the evolution of emotional function.

The major determinants of personality can be viewed as gradations in the intensity of important temperamental characteristics. Mental illnesses like atypical depression result when one of these constitutional propensities rises above a certain threshold of emotional intensity, in response to specific kinds of stress, at which

---

[12] In 2013, the 5th Diagnostic Manual (DSM 5) made both melancholia and atypical depression *specifiers* of the general diagnosis of major depression.

point it escapes its normal regulation and breaks down into feedback reverberation.

Once I saw how clearly atypical depression was related to high levels of separation anxiety, I began to understand the influence of the level of patients' temperamental propensity to separation anxiety on their personalities and how they relate to people around them. I began pointing out the extent to which this one trait was affecting patients' lives in a multiplicity of small ways. In relationships of all kinds, these are the ones most likely to suppress their opinions in order not to break the rapport within the moment. As a result, these people are vulnerable to subtle forms of interpersonal exploitation.

Envisioning the cohering role of separation anxiety in relationships, I found the image of a rubber band helpful as a metaphor for the emotionally aversive component of personal bonds. Separation anxiety exerts a constant, elastic pulling force on relationships between individuals in marriages, families, and friendship ties. It operates at the micro level within personal subgroups as opposed to at the macro, whole-group level, which is where the fear of entrapment, soon to be addressed, operates. So, when I mention the fear of separation as an evolutionary force, think of an aggregate of rubber bands holding individual relationships together within the personally bonded subgroups of a larger group.

Snit disorder

I began my career working in a maximum-security prison. One inmate there, whose countenance still haunts me from time to time, was a gaunt middle-aged man who used to stand in the corner of the common room and blankly stare out the window all day, chain-smoking. His posture, the expression on his face, his movements and gait, all bespoke unrelenting despair. He never talked to anyone, much less to me; but after observing him for a year, I concluded that he was not mentally ill, but that his emotional condition was *existential*.

In psychiatry, we sometimes pluck out complex philosophical concepts and adapt them for our own use, such as our use of phenomenology to refer to the study of subjective symptoms. We call an existential psychiatric condition one that is a direct emotional response to a person's circumstances and is not a sickness. To make such a determination, a judgment must be made about whether the emotional response to a specific set of circumstances is within the normal range of human responses—which is among the most delicate crafts of a psychiatrist. On the fringes of the field of psychiatry there are always those who espouse that all mental illnesses are existential, which is a cruel belief, sustained by ignorance.

At the prison, all the inmates had to attend tier meetings, and he would sit at them week after week, month after month silently staring at the floor. Inexplicably one day, after a long silence, he began to talk, softly, but he could be clearly heard as everyone in the room fell silent and listened intently to what he had to say. Part of what was expected in these meetings was for inmates to walk us through their crimes. He spoke slowly and deliberately with no emotion whatsoever. He'd shot his wife dead one night after drinking. He said he would always love her and was only waiting to die. He then described in spare, clear language how he would enter prolonged periods lasting weeks during which he would be silently enraged at his wife for no apparent reason. She finally told him she couldn't tolerate it anymore and was going to leave him, in response to which he killed her. He said he had been drinking but wanted to make it clear to us that he did not kill her in the heat of an argument. He killed her because he could not stand to be without her. He said he had pleaded guilty and told us he felt he was in the right place. He lapsed back into silence.

In my clinical book, *Diagnosing and Treating Mental Illness*, I describe a common condition that I call *snit disorder*. Snit disorder is a mental state of anger occurring mostly in marriages in which people have high separation sensitivity but also high levels of aggression. Not uncommonly when the relationship is felt to be close, something will happen during a marital interaction that breaks the rapport, such as a careless or unkind comment or even a rejecting gesture. In response, the sufferer is thrown into a state of intense, prolonged rage that can last for days or even weeks. Often the patient might want to rehash the "issue" repeatedly, following the beleaguered spouse around for hours. This is the kind of situation, especially when alcohol is involved, that can lead to spousal abuse.

There are two key factors in the diagnosis of snit disorder. The first, which is the reason I bring it up in this context, is that the individual acutely knows that his (this is mostly a male affliction) anger is being restrained by his separation anxiety. Separation anxiety is dominating overpowering rage. On close analysis, these patients are caught in an emotional feedback loop between their rage, which increases desperate isolation, and separation anxiety, which triggers more "controlling" rage. Whereas most people respond to separation anxiety with anxiety alone, these patients respond to separation anxiety with rage and anxiety. If separation anxiety dominates rage, snit disorder results. If rage overpowers separation anxiety, then the crucial diagnostic criterion of being aware that rage is destructive is not present, and criminal behavior can result. [13]

For these patients, separation anxiety serves as the source of awareness that rage is unreasonable, and yet they are trapped in obsessive thoughts of revenge (fight) and divorce (flight). The other key diagnostic characteristic is that when rage runs its course, extreme remorse, shame, and even humiliation result from the damage wreaked upon the relationship. This state of mind was present in the man described above, and it distinguished him from many other inmates.

In snit disorder, the basic function of separation anxiety comes into focus. Separation anxiety serves to inhibit both the fight and flight responses. Snit disorder takes place almost only in marriages, romantic relationships, and nuclear families, similar to atypical depression. I began to realize that separation anxiety was one of the central emotional forces that, in evolution, tempered the antisocial fight-flight responses, and produced the stable dominance and submission mentalities suitable for group living. Here, buried like a fossil within these individuals, was evidence for a dynamic between separation anxiety and the fight and flight responses that harkened back some 50 million years to group-formation in primates, when that which would make us human first awakened.

Emotional fossils

I had seen that the intense aggression of prison life reveals detailed aspects of the normal social role of aggression. This primed me to recognize that the intense fear of atypical depression also reveals detailed aspects of the normal role of separation anxiety in everyday life. Furthermore, I became convinced that the fact that atypical depression could paralyze all mental function meant that separation anxiety not only occupies a central role in normal psychosocial function, but also played

---

[13] This observation first led me to propose that an essential aspect of conscious self-awareness is the capacity to experience two conflicting emotions simultaneously.

a key role in the deep evolution of our emotions. Can mental illnesses be viewed as emotional fossils?

The original, classical concept of a gene, described by the celebrated work of the Augustinian friar Gregor Mendel (1866), was that it is the indivisible unit of a transmitted genetic recipe, or part thereof for constructing a functioning organism. Although our current understanding is that a gene itself is divisible in many complicated ways, it still retains the aspect of determining a unit of transmitted structure and/or function. Mendel's discovery was that traits are not inherited as continuous gradations but are transmitted within discrete "packets." I propose that the evolution of emotion has similarly taken place by the progressive reconfiguration, over long periods of time, of stable and discrete "bundles" of emotion, such as the fear of separation and the cohering motivation it engenders.

The core idea of an emotional fossil is that mental illnesses reveal these quantum bundles of social emotion and motivation that have remained unchanged, in some instances for hundreds of thousands of years (since the appearance of *Homo sapiens*), and in others, as with separation anxiety, for 52 million years (since group formation in primates). I will also describe how the original primate emotional fossils intensified as part of the evolutionary metamorphosis of apes into hominins six million years ago, which was the single event in the essay's narrative that is most pivotal to how we became human.

Is depression really depression?

There can be two fundamental ways of viewing depression. The most prevalent view is that depression represents the inhibition of goal-directed, pleasure-motivated behavior. For example, there is a section of the rat forebrain (prefrontal cortex) that, when in a chronically hyperactive state, has been demonstrated to downregulate pleasure-motivating areas of the brain (mediated by the neurotransmitter dopamine) and to cause depression-like states (Ferenczi, 2016). However, my discussions with patients with major depressive conditions led me to consider this kind of goal-directed-pleasure-inhibition as secondary to the *hyperactivity of fear-based motivations*.

Note that separation anxiety functions as an aversive motivation. Anxiety is a painful emotion and, as with physical pain, avoidance is the motivation that is engendered by it. As just mentioned, we assume that motivation involves the seeking of pleasure, but much of our social behavior is directed by the avoidance of painful feelings. Patients with deficits in the ability to experience physical pain constantly injure themselves, and those with deficits in experiencing social pain injure others.

The brain is mainly an inhibitory organ. If the more recently evolved structures, such as the outer cortex, are severed from the more interior ancient structures, the muscles of the entire body lock down into a state of violent tonic contraction called *opisthotonos*. Similarly, separation anxiety, as is plainly illustrated in snit disorder, normally inhibits and regulates the more ancient and socially disruptive impulses of fight and flight. So along with being experienced as painful, an intrinsic function of separation anxiety is that it inhibits and is in a state of dynamic balance with other emotions and motivations.

I clearly remember a conversation with a patient with persistent atypical depression triggered by rejection from a romantic relationship. I made an observation, which would thenceforth be repeated many times, that had far-reaching consequences for how I view mental illnesses in general. In her mind, she obsessively immersed herself in images of idealized romantic experiences she'd had with him. As she entered into and out of these vivid memory states of reunion, her anxiety was momentarily relieved, but then doubly re-exacerbated by being dragged back into the painful reality of her separated status. The obsessive remembering is like an addictive, short-acting drug that whipped her back and forth such that she was torturing herself—but could not stop. In this process, her separation anxiety was placed into a tight little closed-loop feedback circuit that pathologically intensified it, which I came to identify as the core of the illness.

These mental states are driven by feedback reverberation between complete immersion into a *relational* mentality, and her *own* anxious reaction to it. This concept of separation anxiety transforming into atypical depression by entering a reverberating circuit that pathologically intensifies this anxiety was to influence my understanding of all mental illnesses.

However, the symptoms that designate a condition as depression are lethargy and lack of initiative known as *anergy* (no energy) along with the inability to experience pleasure known as *anhedonia*. This same patient had classical signs of atypical depression: she could hardly get up in the morning, having zero initiative to do anything but lie in bed. One day, while in my office, her ex-boyfriend paged her, and she asked me to allow her to call him from my office. He had decided to get back together with her while she was right in front of me! It was not surprising that it elated her, but what struck me was the magnitude of her physical transformation. She went from the proverbial sack of potatoes to being vibrant in a matter of minutes. The principal question then became the causal relationship between the so-called *negative* anergic symptoms and what I was now conceiving as the core problem of pathologically hyperactive separation anxiety. I decided that (the illness of) depression is really not depression (the symptoms of anergy and anhedonia).

There are two explanations for the anergic symptoms. First, the intrinsic inhibitory property of separation anxiety itself greatly intensifies in such a way as to cause a massive and global inhibition of all emotions, or, second, at a certain threshold of anxious intensity, a brain-mediated *shut-down* mechanism is elicited in response. Perhaps this physical shut-down response evolved to protect the sufferer from the intolerable screaming pitch of sustained states of anxiety—which is possibly an adaptation evolved to protect the sufferer from suicide.

Theoretically, if the anergic symptoms are the result of the inhibitory aspect of pathologically intense anxiety, the patient would be locked into a state of excruciating mental catatonia analogous to the tonic muscular contraction of opisthotonos. Indeed, this kind of emotional catatonia is seen in atypical depression (and more in melancholic depression and even more so in schizophrenia). In *The Noonday Demon: An Atlas of Depression* (2001), which is a lavish gift of sympathy to those who suffer from depression, Andrew Solomon describes his own experience with depression precipitated by the breakup of a romantic relationship. Note how his fear paralyzes him:

> Depression minutes are like dog years, based on some artificial notion of time. I can remember lying frozen in bed, crying because I was too frightened to take a shower, and at the same time knowing that showers are not scary. I kept running through the individual steps in my mind: you turn and put your feet on the floor; you stand; you walk from here to the bathroom; you open the bathroom door; you walk to the edge of the tub; you turn on the water; you step under the water; you rub yourself with soap; you rinse; you step out; you dry yourself; you walk back to the bed. Twelve steps, which sounded to me as onerous as a tour through the stations of the cross.

However, in many patients, the element of fear is in the background and the anergic symptoms predominate. As I observed that patients with atypical depression in on-and-off relationships alternate in and out of a state of illness, I was nudged in the direction that the anergic symptoms were a separate brain-shut-down reaction in response to the hyperactive anxiety.

In addition, I consulted on a handful of hospitalized patients overwhelmed by systemic infections. The families were concerned at the degree of their patient-relatives' lethargy and utter lack of initiative. I ended up reassuring these families that this was a normal, self-protective mental shut-down mechanism that would remit in accordance with improvement in the infectious condition, which invariably proved to be the case.

I decided there was evidence for both mechanisms. For my primary purpose here of targeting stigma, it does not matter whether the anergy is an intrinsic part of the emotional hyperactivity or a secondary reaction to it (like the relationship between a fever and an infection). In both instances the important insight for this essay is that, although the obvious symptoms of depression are most often anergic (from which these conditions draw their name), the actual pathology lies in the sustained magnitude of intense states of anxiety.

Therefore, in my search for the evolutionary meaning of depression and other mental illnesses, I could disregard all anergic symptoms as secondary and reactive to the core of the pathology that existed as white-hot caldrons of emotion radiating inner fragments of the nature of our nature.

I had additional reasons for arriving at this crucial conclusion.

Drug studies

I cannot overstate the impact of the introduction of Prozac in 1987 on shifting attitudes toward mental illness. Almost overnight, mental illness became a "chemical imbalance" (brain disorder) and "all in the genes" rather than a disorder of mental function. I became fascinated by the effects of Prozac and began asking patients to give detailed descriptions of how it altered their emotional experience. I concluded that it decreases people's emotional reactivity to their lives: "My children were driving me crazy and my boss is a yeller. Since taking Prozac, it all just doesn't get to me as much." A New York City friend called me one night from Madison Square Garden during a Knicks game, upset that Prozac had turned him into an "out-of-towner": no hysterics at the slam dunks.

As already stated, I realized that the core pathological process evident in the *experience* of mental illness is the loss of regulation of specific key emotions, which results in their unrestrained release into pathological hyperactivity. I concluded that all medical psychiatric treatments (as opposed to psychotherapy—which probably, to a degree, has this same effect) amounted to "turning the emotional volume down."

Over the years, I have found several studies (Sakin, 1999; Azuma, 2007) supporting the idea that electroconvulsive treatment (ECT) for depression is effective because of the inhibitory phase after the massive stimulation of an induced convulsive seizure. Indeed, some think that deep brain stimulation is effective by interrupting the hyperactivity of a chronically overactive area in the frontal lobe (Mayberg, 2005).

Taking a wider view, new evidence has confirmed what I have already stated: that the higher, more recently evolved brain structures in the outer cortex are in an inhibitory relationship with the primary emotions that spring from the far more ancient brain centers lower down (Northoff et al, 2009). It is important in understanding clinical depression that these conditions involve varieties of inhibitory emotion, such as separation anxiety, that escape into pathological hyperactivity to cause the experience of mental illness. The basic impulse/experience of fear emits from ancient strata of the brain, but its specificity for separation and, its capacity for exquisitely sensitive up-and-down social modulation would be the more recently evolved capacities that have played a central role in how we became human.

I realize that I am making sweeping claims about the nature of mental illness, but I remind you that we are investigating the experiential dimension. As noted in the introduction, this essay is a blending of the scientific method with the empathic method—and with the urgent purpose of eradicating stigma. Accordingly, both reason and empathy are required to judge whether this unfolding evolutionary narrative quickens our ancestors' bones and stones with ancient sensibilities excavated from their hidden legacy inside our own minds by the experience of mental illness.

My aim is to humanize mental illness by providing a framework to enable authentic empathy with what they experience, while making crystal clear that the sheer magnitude of their suffering, recognizable as it may be, sets them apart, and that they abundantly deserve the care and harmony that is our duty to those afflicted with these overwhelming illnesses.

It appears to me that the mechanism of mental illness is like cancer, in which the inhibitory regulation on the growth of cells fails;[14] but the primary events that initiate psychiatric pathology are not genetic mutations that occur at the biochemical level as they are in cancer.

You are now well acquainted with the general pathological mechanism of feedback reverberation. On the Fourth of July, the politician gets up on the podium and tries to begin his speech. Suddenly there is a piercing squeal from the speakers that only gets worse. The sound of his voice enters the microphone, is amplified, emerges from the speaker, and then is picked up through the overly sensitive microphone; repeating this circuit builds into an escalating screech in an instant. Either a sound barrier needs to be placed between the microphone and the speaker, or the volume must be turned down so the microphone can no longer pick up its own output. I became convinced that psychiatric medications, such as Prozac, effectively "turn down the volume" of hyperactive emotions such that they can slip back into their properly regulated function.

Each of the social emotions, such as separation anxiety, are experienced in the mind as the result of diffusively complex physiological processes at the brain level. However, the subjective experience of pathology in atypical depression (the mind level) is comprised of feedback reverberation between two mind states: the emotional memory of a now lost relational experience, and the patient's escalating, real-time response of separation anxiety in reaction to it, which then bids back the feeling-laden relational memories even stronger. Prozac clearly helps slow feedback reverberation down, but the take-home point here is that the actual pathology is happening at the level of the mind.

Having discussed the relationship between the experience of atypical depression and normally functioning separation anxiety, the next chapter will undertake an evolutionary psychoanalysis of melancholia.

---

[14] Decreased cell death (*apoptosis*) is also a factor in cancer (Brown, 2005).

CHAPTER 4

ENTRAPMENT AND BANISHMENT

Melancholia

Beginning in 1975 I hospitalized my patients on a psychiatric unit located on the seventh floor of Sibley Memorial Hospital in Washington, D.C., where I served for a term as chair of the department. Shortly after the wing opened in 1961, a large, muscular patient ran the length of the lounge area in full view of everyone and flew headfirst with his arms down at one of the picture windows, shattering it and plunging to his death six stories below. By the time I worked at Sibley, the windows had been replaced with impenetrable tempered glass. The next patient who attempted to "spear" himself through a window on Seven West left some hair stuck in a starburst pattern of cracked glass. I am not sure what these two patients' diagnoses were, but such behavior would be consistent with agitated melancholic depression.

Melancholia is one of the most dreaded of all mental illnesses. Aptly named by Hippocrates, melancholia means black bile, which remains a potent metaphor for the interior experience of this dreadful condition. Someone enveloped by atypical depression is often receptive and can find a reprieve from suffering in the offerings of warmth and personal support from others. In stark contrast, there is no amnesty to be had from melancholia, in which the blackness of the mood derives from a total preoccupation with escape into oblivion and nothingness: "I feel dead; my life is over."

The fundamental difference between the two poles of melancholic depression and atypical depression can be appreciated through a close examination of suicidal intent in both. In atypical depression, the issue is not so much escape from the pain of the current circumstance as it is focused on reunion with a lost person, even at the expense of self-destructive behavior. Not uncommonly, a suicide attempt in these patients is a desperate attempt to have a rejecting person rescue him or at least pay attention to his suffering in a sometimes-fatal failure of judgment. Similarly, in pathological grief reactions, thoughts of suicide take the form of rejoining the deceased person.

In melancholia, the alternative of death, or simply "not existing," is an intrinsic part of the condition—not as a positive place to go, but rather as an escape from the intolerable current subjective experience. Whereas in atypical depression, the person yearns and reaches for memories in the past of something lost, the focus in melancholia is a sudden loss of hope for the future, a sense of being intolerably trapped within the excruciating present with the only definitive escape being death. Seeking an escape from an intense feeling of entrapment is as intrinsic to melancholic depression as seeking a reconnection from separation in atypical depression.

The importance of escape to the condition of melancholia revealed itself in the many interactions I had while initiating and maintaining hospitalization for these tortured patients. Hospitalization at Sibley's psychiatric unit has always been voluntary. All the patients I admitted to this unit had to sign themselves in. I remember one in particular.

I am sitting in a small room in the admitting area of the hospital. The patient is accompanied by his spouse and general physician. The patient has been talking incessantly about committing suicide for a week, and his wife and PCP have convinced him to come this far. A consent form is on the table in front of him. He himself knows he needs the protection of the hospital. But he cannot bring himself to sign the form. He cannot bear the thought of forgoing the one reliable access to escaping the hell he is experiencing. His mind is not preoccupied by the process of suicide itself, but by escape—the relief it represents.

Assuming the authority of healer, I convey by implication my determination relentlessly to face down the alien force that possesses his mind. Nested within the sternness of this posture, I address the patient as the helpless hostage he knows in his heart of hearts he is. I reassure him I have tools well up to subduing the powerful sickness that torments him, and then resume my steely opposition to the soulless foe in possession of his mind. His wife is holding his hand lovingly. His physician tells him I am right. He picks up the pen and is about to sign his name, but then he puts it down. He is not ready yet. I reveal not the slightest twinge of frustration; I was expecting it and persist—and eventually succeed. Long after he is cured, in a follow-up office visit he and his wife recall my intervention with gratitude, and I am moved. Patients rarely wish to recall such painful events once they recede.

After the patient signed into the psychiatric unit at Sibley, I had the legal authority to hold him against his will for 48 hours from the time of his request to be discharged. After two days elapsed, I had to decide whether I considered the patient "an immediate threat to him/herself or others." If I thought the patient posed such a threat, it was then my duty to file a "petition," along with another physician, to compel the patient to undergo a psychiatric examination at *another* institution to determine the need for further detention; but this commitment procedure could be initiated only after the patient left Sibley Hospital! Thank goodness I never had to resort to such a convoluted process.

At one time in my life, as with many busy mental health practitioners, it was part of my daily routine to be in bare-knuckle adversarial negotiations with several individuals in passionate advocacy for the continuation of their very existence. Inevitably the issue came down to the patient's desperate determination to hold on to access to the option of committing suicide. Consider a state of mind in which, although physically healthy, you feel so trapped in despair that all you can think about is escaping into death. Now imagine that in such a state of mind you have voluntarily placed yourself in the psychiatric unit of a hospital where it is nearly impossible to commit suicide. The doctor is making rounds every day and talking to you in the attempt to ascertain whether you would commit suicide if discharged.

You, the patient, are placed in the position such that all you have to do is to pretend to be healthy to fool the doctor into releasing you, so you can go out and destroy yourself. But when you are in the grip of melancholia, you cannot fake mental equilibrium any more than you can fake happiness when a loved one has just died. The very definition of mental illness is to be in a mental state in which emotions are so intense that they control thoughts and behavior. This was a high-stakes cat-and-mouse game in which my only credibility was the degree to which I could authentically assume the ancient role of healer. The patient's family was always heavily involved in these decisions. My stance was unambiguously simple: Your mind is in the grip of a sickness distorting your emotions and, as a direct result, your beliefs and motivations. I cannot recall a situation in which I kept someone in the hospital when it turned out not to have been justified, as portrayed in the popular 1975 movie *One Flew Over the Cuckoo's Nest*, which trivializes the suffering I am describing.

Just as every doctor loses patients to illness, every psychiatrist, including myself, loses patients to suicide; each haunts me. A half dozen shot themselves, one threw himself into The Great Falls of the Potomac River, and one drank a gallon of antifreeze. Terrible ignominy surrounds a suicide from melancholic illness in friends and relatives of the deceased patient, including, of course, the psychiatrist. It should not be so, but there it is. Suicide leaves behind the most intense feelings of guilt I have ever experienced, while fully understanding that the survivors' pain, does not approach the emotional intensity of melancholia itself. Even though these deaths are caused by a disease endemic to our human nature, there is nothing natural about suicide in the perception of others when it happens.

I began practicing hospital psychiatry before insurance companies began funding only very short hospital stays. It was not unusual for a patient with melancholia to spend a month or two in the hospital, with medications not as advanced as they are today. Back then, it became clear to me in following the progress of these desperately suicidal patients through long hospital visits that the "trap" represented by being confined to the hospital desensitized them to the feeling of entrapment that was the very essence of their illness. Being able to relax within the confines of the hospital psychiatric unit and to participate in its lively social milieu diminished, by proxy, the intense feelings of entrapment that had originally made up their emotional illness. Once the feeling of being trapped had evaporated, so did all the motivations and rationales that had been constructed in response to such an overwhelming emotion.

A moving and articulate firsthand account of melancholia is the short memoir *Darkness Visible* (1990) by William Styron, celebrated author of *Sophie's Choice*:

> . . . it is not an immediately identifiable pain, like that of a broken limb. It may be more accurate to say that despair, owing to some evil trick played upon the sick brain by the inhabiting psyche, comes to resemble the diabolical discomfort of being imprisoned in a fiercely over-heated room. And because no breeze stirs this caldron, because there is no escape from this smothering confinement, it is entirely natural that the victim begins to think ceaselessly of oblivion.

After the failure of multiple modalities of psychiatric treatment, Styron finally healed in the course of a lengthy hospitalization.

Having observed early in my career that melancholia involved intense feelings of entrapment and the resulting need for escape, at times via suicide, I pondered the meaning of these symptoms for many years. When I concluded that atypical depression involved the shut-down symptoms of lack of initiative and will, I noted that these symptoms were also embedded in melancholia.

I have discussed my deliberations on the role of the low-energy symptoms in atypical depression as to whether it was a shut-down reaction or a freeze response to the core intense anxiety. I noted that the anergic shut-down symptoms in melancholia seemed far more engaged with the core hyperactive pathology than in atypical depression. Past a point of no return in melancholia, the paralysis of willpower itself engenders the terror of being trapped by the inability to initiate behavior of any sort. The fear of being trapped rises to a threshold beyond which the paralysis engendered by this fear itself increases to a sustained high pitch. The more terrified of entrapment one becomes, the more paralysis sets in, resulting in the collapse of towering frustration into the groundlessness of despair. There ensues the locking down into a frozen, vicious cycle of the agony of being trapped by one's emotional paralysis.

The drug curare paralyzes all muscular movement by inactivating the nerves at their peripheral *end plate* juncture with all the voluntary muscles. Curare is used in surgery after the administration of a general anesthetic to obtain complete relaxation of the musculature. Imagine how it would feel to be given curare without the unconsciousness induced by the anesthetic. Perhaps a better comparison of how melancholia feels would be to imagine this experience from the point of view of the muscles themselves, severed from all communication from their brain.

The fear of entrapment

Vivid images conveying the fear of being trapped were captured in certain horrifying images on September 11, 2001, at the World Trade Center. The entire nation was gripped by the sight of desperately trapped people leaning away from a raging fire from shattered windows, many eventually flinging themselves out with their downtown suits streaming upward, neckties like tiny banners.

I have come to understand from my patients with melancholia that we all emotionally experience our societies as vertical funnels that threaten to entrap us below but that open as we ascend, according to a broad variety of parameters. The direction of all economic and work life in general is upward from beneath. The fundamental motivation of work is to labor in the deeply felt direction of less and less social constriction. Most people get up and go to work in the morning not because they want to, but because they are afraid of what will happen if they do not. In contrast, ambition is both a goal-and-future-oriented motivation, which is wholly different and will be discussed in Chapter 9. Suffice it to say for now that, in the dimension of time, melancholia is experienced as the imposition of an intolerable social claustrophobia produced by the sudden evaporation of all ambition. The future completely disappears, and all hope along with it.

Melancholia does not appear out of nowhere. There might be an unexpected reversal usually in the general area of one's work life. Business is suddenly down, a mistake is made, there is some half-step backward enough to dissolve the salutary effects of social productivity that neutralized the anxiety of being trapped. Perhaps it is the suddenness of the reappearance of this anxiety—to a threshold at which the feedback reverberation of mental illness sets in—that then triggers the same shut-down mechanisms described in atypical depression.

Because the shut-down response is a more intrinsic part of the pathology in melancholia than in atypical depression, it is more intractable. While atypical depression usually involves the loss of just one person, melancholia is experienced as a global social degradation that cannot be penetrated by sympathy from friends. Elicited by intense feelings of shame, the shut-down response contributes to an excruciating feeling of being paralyzed by one's utter lack of any initiative whatsoever. Is it somehow possible that an evolved shut-down response could be protecting the person from committing suicide even as it aggravates the intolerable anxiety of being trapped?

Social claustrophobia

Phobias are conditions in which specific circumstances elicit panic. Common phobias are fear of heights, crowds, bridges, dogs, and cars. The list is endless; just place the feared object or situation in front of the suffix phobia, and you have the diagnosis. One of the most common is claustrophobia, which is the fear of being trapped in enclosed spaces. Unlike many phobias, claustrophobia clearly has adaptive evolutionary roots. A cornered animal becomes dangerous because it panics. It is reasonable that the atavistic fear of being trapped in the physical environment was commandeered—a process called *exaptation*—during the evolution of sociality beginning about 52 million years ago when primates began forming groups.

Decades ago, I saw an able young woman seeking treatment for claustrophobia. She'd been born into difficult circumstances, and her efforts to escape her past were rewarded thanks to the time-tested combination of hard work and talent. This woman's socially upward momentum toward greater freedom was suddenly blocked by a failure at work, and in addition, she said she felt trapped within a romantic relationship.

One day as she stood in a crowded New York subway station, a train came roaring in and she panicked. If you have not had this New York City experience, it is like being a spark plug in the crankcase cylinder of a truck while the piston is hurtling down at you. The approaching train is very loud and screechy, with an end-of-the-world crescendo of sound right before it quickly diminishes and stops.

Thereafter, this person became claustrophobic about being in elevators, theaters, restaurants, and other enclosed spaces. I told her that her heightened concerns about being socially trapped in her life (stifled ambition) had been transformed into physical claustrophobia. I pointed out that she had been supersaturated with the ambient fear of being socially trapped, which was then precipitated into physical claustrophobia by the subway train (regressed back into its pre-social function). She agreed with my analysis, but as is often the case, while such interpretations may give patients a sense of orientation about their condition, the interpretations do not affect the symptoms. Besides discussing her social circumstances at length, I treated her phobia by encouraging a combination of graduated exposure to claustrophobic circumstances that desensitized her anxious reactions plus small doses of targeted tranquilizing medication.

This woman's transformation from a mood to a phobic fear revealed similarities between the two. In phobias, the fear is caused by a physically external circumstance and the response is to avoid it. Prior to the phobia, this woman's depressed mood (which was existential and not pathological) was also a response to external circumstances, but these were social circumstances in which she was embedded and not so easily avoided. The principal insight illustrated in melancholia is that, although moods appear to be our most personal inner environment, close examination of their subjective experience reveal them to be a response to the social environment. A primary behavior of the depressed person is to withdraw socially, perhaps like the response in a phobia to something inanimate, or even worse, to a spider—which brings me the crucial point that in melancholia, the social environment is felt to be an *active agent* intentionally inflicting feelings of depression, resulting in the emotions of guilt and shame.

Where does guilt and shame come from?

Shame is an inherently collective emotion that requires a shaming "audience" socially condemning the person, whereas guilt is a private, internal affair in which an action is the focus. In melancholia there can be obsessive guilt about specific acts, but melancholia is driven by the experience of social condemnation.

Freudian psychoanalytic interpretations of the origins of guilt and shame entail an emotional reversal in the developing child's mind that results in the child's anger turning inward. This inward-directed anger forms the foundation of a normally functioning superego that modulates the sexual and aggressive strivings of the id, and this process is pathologically exaggerated in melancholic depression.

One day, while listening to a patient suffering from melancholia talk about his distorted beliefs about other people's negative attitudes toward him, I thought to myself, *What if this patient is correctly perceiving that the source of his melancholia, and the accompanying guilt and shame, actually is, in some manner, emanating from the social sphere?* For many years I had thought that mental illnesses were the pathological intensification of normal emotional functions. Freud himself thought that unconscious guilt is part of a normally functioning superego. But Freud was thinking in the paradigm of the individual patient's childhood development, and I had become immersed in the evolution of our species.

Evolutionary developmental biology (evo-devo) is a field that explores how the developmental processes of organisms themselves evolve. From a Freudian standpoint the oedipal drama *internalizes* the child's fear of retaliation for jealous anger toward a parent, which then is distilled into the guilt and shame of the developing superego. The simplest evolutionary explanation of this developmental transformation of the child's anger invokes the most controversial of all of Darwin's theories: *group selection*. Here I introduce this fraught topic with much more to follow. The process of natural selection occurring at the level of groups expands the scope of the arena from the life of a child to the evolution of childhood development through deep time.

On the grand stage of evolution, the child's oedipal drama has been choreographed by the life force of natural selection to serve the interests of the group and not the child. So, when that patient perceived the source of guilt and shame to be the social environment, he was not just projecting his own anger; this anger had been vouchsafed to the social sphere since childhood as part of his evolutionary legacy as a human being. The superego was not instilled into the child's mind, the child's mind was instilled into the collective social mind.

 It is useful to become familiar with the concept of *intentionality*, which has to do with a defining quality of mind that involves direction and agency: all minds are characterized by agency, or willfulness, directed at some object or circumstance. I propose that the social/relational sphere possesses these essential qualities required to be considered within the category of mind, albeit a collective one. The word 'intentionality' is needed to express this counterintuitive idea that human groups themselves (networks of relationships as a whole) evolved to possess the quality of agency and direction, and this direction is experienced as squarely aimed at the individuals within a group.

Replicating every generation, the collective emotions and motivations in networks of hominin relationships over the eons have been submitted to the functional molding of natural selection for the benefits of *teamwork* (much more on this to come), and this process has left the instinctual residue of collective intentionality embedded in the social sphere of humans. These are the seeds of the spiritual in Darwin's idea.

The hypothesis that shame and guilt are aversive motivations that are naturally selected to emanate from groups to promote their survival-by-cohesion is the most simple and parsimonious explanation for the evolution of the superego. Constrained by individual-only evolutionary thinking, the superego would have had to arise by means of contorted, competitive survival strategies between individuals akin to honor among thieves. This is not an important clinical distinction, but philosophically, in relation to what constitutes our human nature, the idea that the superego was evolved collectively at the level of groups is immense.

The fear of banishment

From my patients, I picture the melancholic circumstance conferred by the emotions experienced in melancholia as not only entrapment at the periphery of society, but also standing on the precipice of banishment. The psychoanalytic term for such a connected dyad of emotions is a *complex*. The two fears of this complex of being trapped and banished, although now bound together in us, each probably evolved by different mechanisms, and at very different periods of our evolutionary history.

Likely, the dawn of group association among primates some 52 million years ago was accompanied by an increase in separation anxiety among blood relatives; separation anxiety promoting close associations would have been derived from mammalian emotions inherent to the mother–infant bond, along with positive feelings of physical closeness emphasized by Freud. Selected for the benefits of group association, separation anxiety must have spread from the mother-infant bond to wider kinship groups, forming a key motivational ingredient of *kin selection*.

Connected to this early process, it is logical to propose that natural selection for the survival of groups commandeered (exapted) from individuals the atavistic fear of physical entrapment into the fear of social entrapment at the bottom or periphery of groups. Note that the feeling of entrapment provoked by low status in the hierarchical structure of primate groups is caused by a social circumstance external to the individual, similar to claustrophobia, but, in this case, the fear emanates from the felt outer edges that define the experience of a group.

The sense of banishment manifested in melancholia goes beyond the experience of being trapped at the periphery of one's hierarchy (as in poverty) to include the distinct sensibility that the surrounding social environment is justifiably condemning the patient for *wrongdoing*, causing intense feelings of shame. In this aspect of melancholia, one's social group and society at large become active agents emitting vague accusations at the beleaguered individual. I assumed that this same experience of society plays an intentional role in normal social interactions, albeit in a far more attenuated and unconscious manner. I have concluded that the transformation of the social sphere into an active, intentional agent is a hallmark of our entire hominin tribe. A plausible pathway to such a transformation in our earliest ancestral species is the central topic in Chapter 7, titled "A New Form of Life."

Here is yet another example of a mental illness revealing important aspects of our emotions that are concealed during their muted normal function. Our lives are lived within worlds of collective moods created by our associations, not only in our personal relationships but also in our affiliation with the larger groups in which we dwell. Without being aware of it, we all live within a centripetal emotional *force field* comprised of social claustrophobia elicited by entrapment at the periphery of our groups where banishment is possible.

The paradox in the depressive mood disorders, particularly notable in melancholia, is that from the outside the suffering appears to be a completely private hell, but from the inside this experience is embedded in an actively humiliating social circumstance. Overwhelmingly negative feelings are focused on the individual as if a fetid, paralytic poison (black bile) is being secreted into the person from the social sphere.

Could it be that the moods that we daily experience as our innermost feelings actually radiate from the intentions of the nested groups in which we all find ourselves immersed? Could it be that our moods are the echoes of an ancient willfulness that has surrounded us as a living ark within which we have sought shelter, huddled together with one another, through the countless storms of our tumultuous voyage down through the eons?

Note to clinicians. As you well know, symptoms of these two poles of depression often present as blended combinations in a single patient, as are mixed symptoms of schizophrenia and bipolar disorder common. Such clinical complexities go beyond the scope of this essay.

CHAPTER 5

TRAPPED AND STRANDED

Panic

An endearing, entertaining young woman first presented herself in my office in a state of extreme distress. Kathy wanted to be an elementary school teacher, and she enrolled in an apprentice program that placed her as an assistant teacher at an inner-city school. Because she was white and middle-class, she felt that the predominantly African American administration looked upon her two-year commitment there with some skepticism. But she loved working with the children and had a gift for relating to them.

However, some of these kids had tough circumstances at home, and they brought these problems to school, resulting in continual dramas of sorting out conflicts. Because of events that remained unclear in her mind, she was shocked to be called into the principal's office and told that a student had accused her of something she did not do.

Kathy could easily be a successful stand-up comedian. She is the kind of person driven to entertain whoever she was with. But at that time, I saw in her deep concern that anyone would suspect her of the accusation made against her—and the problem was not going away. She knew by the principal's attitude that she had not dismissed the possibility that Kathy may have been guilty. After Kathy was placed on probation, she was unable to tolerate the suspicion now reinforced. She had embraced a future of teaching children and was eager to begin her training in the toughest kind of situation. But now she encountered a toxic atmosphere. Her first panic episodes were accompanied by a suffocating sensation, causing her to gasp for air. When she burst into my office, she asked repeatedly, "Dr. Wylie, am I going crazy? Please tell me whether I am going crazy."[15]

The linking of two social emotions

Almost invariably present in the early experience of pathological panic is the sensation of suffocation, technically called *air hunger*. With the onset of a panic episode, patients cannot get enough air in their lungs and begin gasping. Clearly there is feedback reverberation between the physical sensation of suffocation and the anxiety in response to it. In addition, hyperventilation causes lightheadedness and tingling in the extremities and around the mouth; these are the effects of low carbon dioxide, which is excessively exhaled. These physical symptoms can be reversed by breathing into a paper bag to rebreathe CO_2. Well, it turns out that carbon dioxide levels are involved on a far deeper level than the paper bag maneuver would imply.

In 1984, psychiatrist Jack Gorman and his colleagues at Columbia first demonstrated that patients with panic disorder have a higher sensitivity to increased levels of carbon dioxide.[16] This prompted research on precipitating panic attacks in the laboratory by the controlled administration of CO_2. In 1993, Donald Klein, who was a coauthor of the Gorman paper and also at Columbia, published a paper titled "False Suffocation Alarms, Spontaneous Panics, and Related Conditions: An Integrated Approach." Based on these laboratory studies, Klein proposed that carbon dioxide hypersensitivity in the brain stem area made these patients vulnerable to "*false* suffocation alarms," namely, panic attacks; that this was probably inheritable; and that it was the root cause of panic disorder. In addition, he thought antidepressants were effective in controlling panic disorder because they desensitized carbon dioxide receptors in the brain stem.

---

[15] Here *crazy* is used appropriately to refer to the radical alteration of normalcy that is characteristic of major mental illness with a genuine expression of fear no different than that of, say, cancer.

[16] This could explain why panic attacks can occur during sleep, when CO_2 levels can be high. Also, theoretically, this would mean that overdoing the paper bag maneuver could make matters worse.

Klein's paper was published at the height of the initial surge in the biological revolution in psychiatry away from the dominance of psychoanalytic ideas. When Dr. Klein came to Washington to give a talk on the subject, I remember his intense enthusiasm about hard evidence that a major psychiatric illness had a bona fide physical cause.[17]

However, I was already committed to a whole different level of causality—that of natural selection. Claustrophobia is associated with CO_2 sensitivity (air hunger) as part of a fight-flight response to cope with physical entrapment. However, when physical claustrophobia was commandeered (exapted) to serve group formation, perhaps its associated CO_2 sensitivity was exapted as method to *ramp up* social claustrophobia. Thus CO_2 sensitivity transformed from triggering physical claustrophobia to a way natural selection for the benefits of the group "mind" could increase sensitivity to social claustrophobia. Evolution by natural selection works by taking whatever raw materials are available, in this case physical claustrophobia and CO_2 sensitivity, and alters them it in ways that are adaptive, in this case to the survival of groups.

By talking to patients with panic disorder over the years, I noted that physical sensations of suffocation were only the endpoint on a continuum of a more general fear of being trapped. For example, patients with panic disorder generally do not like hot weather, which they experience as confining, "like a wet blanket covering me." Most decisive was the observation that the circumstances surrounding the initial episodes of panic invariably involved these patients feeling themselves, even without being aware of it, to be in an entrapped situation, like the circumstances of the woman in whom claustrophobia was precipitated in the New York subway station.

Increased brain receptor sensitivity triggers a sensation of suffocation evolved to be elicited by circumstances in which individuals find themselves coerced toward

---

[17] There is an extra incentive for psychiatrists to find biological causes for mental illnesses to counteract a substantial antipsychiatry opinion that mental illnesses do not really exist. On the other hand, this same incentive may lead *bottom-up* investigators who are looking for causes in the biochemistry or genetics of the brain to dismiss *top-down* explanations for mental illness, such as those presented in this book.

the periphery of a social group. In Kathy's case, her group was the school in which she worked and the teaching profession in general.

I had already conceived that a major factor in hominin evolution over six million years was a marked strengthening of group bonds, which I then felt was an avoidance response to the intensified sensitivity to suffocation elicited by being trapped at the periphery of one's groups. Perhaps panic disorder sufferers in general are simply out on the more sensitive end of a bell curve that has generally been shifted decisively in the direction of an increase in this specific sensitivity, not just in modern humans but in our entire hominin tribe.

Apart from the physical symptom of suffocation, the most prominent symptom in panic disorder is the fear of "going crazy." That was Kathy's continuing concern for many weeks and months; after her first experience of panic she needed constant reassurance that she was not psychotic. I had noted this fear countless times previously in panic disorder patients and had examined and considered it carefully. I arrived at the hypothesis that the primary fear of suffocation, which I felt to be an intense feeling of being trapped, caused the patient to escape this intolerable feeling by distancing him/herself from it psychologically.

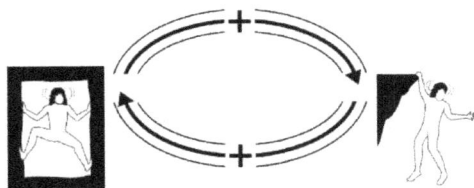

However, this produced an equally frightening feeling of self-separation, technically called *depersonalization*, in which the sufferer experiences a weird, disconnected feeling state that then elicits a frantic fear of going psychotic. I hypothesized that the self-sustaining aspect of panic disorder was a rapid oscillation (feedback reverberation) between psychological escape from suffocation into a state of depersonalization, back and forth. So the "panic" in clinical panic disorder is a debilitating, species-specific (except for dogs) variety of panic involving a relapsing pathological interaction between the fears discussed in the last two chapters.

Too gentle?

There was another aspect to Kathy's situation. If a group of people lined up according to the degree they were out for themselves as individuals, the looking-out-for-number-one types on one end, and the for-the-good-of-the-group types whose instincts tend toward selflessness on the other end, the panic disorder patients generally fall into the latter group. It is as if they are given an extra dose of that which benefits groups, in contrast to the characteristics that make up those who are primarily concerned with their own goals. Kathy certainly fit the former mold, which was one reason her predicament was upsetting in the first place. She was not the kind of person who would engage in whatever she had been accused of. Sometimes our sessions would end up with Kathy entertaining me with her comedic talents, as it was part of her instinct to be sensitive to and care for others.

She suffered terribly and needed real help, which meant medications. I prescribe for her varieties of medication to subdue anxiety, which would calm her down to a point. But then the difficulty of her circumstance would flare, and her panic would break through the buffering effect of the medication. The pathology of her fear metastasized into including the teaching circumstance in general, and when the term ended, she decided to end her dream of becoming a teacher. The thought of walking into a classroom full of kids now was simply too frightening.

Cruelly, once panic establishes itself in a patient's brain, the patient is forever more prone to relapse, and relapse Kathy did, for many years afterward. She moved to Florida; I assume to get far away. She continued to call me from time to time. She became a personal trainer but continued to be plagued by panic episodes, for example when she was "trapped" by a client for the period of the appointment. Her efforts at establishing close relationships were also affected because they represented traps and would precipitate panic episodes.

In Frans de Waal's first popular book, *Chimpanzee Politics* (1982), he writes:

> I clearly remember the first dream I had about chimpanzees. In it my preoccupation with the distance between them and me was apparent. During this dream the large door to their quarters was opened for me from the inside. The apes were pushing each other aside in order to get a good look at me. Yeron, the oldest male, stepped forward and shook my hand. Rather impatiently he listened to my request to come in. He refused point blank. That was out of the

question, he said, and besides, their society would not suit me: it was much too harsh for a human being.

I, too, concluded that the direction of hominin evolution is toward greater gentleness and that patients suffer from the ultra-sensitivity of their temperaments, which constituted the susceptibility to panic disorder.[18] I hypothesized that the fears of separation and entrapment evolved right at the beginning of group formation in primates some 52 million years ago, but now I suspected that the intensification of those fears was an intrinsic feature of the evolutionary transition from apes to hominins.

The fear of being trapped extends to all aspects of social life. One can feel trapped in poverty, low social status, a dead-end job, or a romantic relationship, but at the same time one can be afraid to separate from the sense of security these circumstances engender. These two anxieties hang in the balance within every single social contact. To feel these fears, to struggle with them daily and work through them with measured steps, is part of being human—and especially of being young. Life is often a struggle between bondage and loneliness.

It is as if panic disorder patients develop an allergy to life itself. They experience these emotions acutely and show us plainly how we all feel. They have been chosen for their immense honesty and humanity, daily forced to wrestle life right down at the bare roots of what it is.

I have presented experiential evidence from melancholia that social emotions evolved to emanate from the groups in which we live. In the following chapter the evolutionary significance of schizophrenia, the most mysterious of all maladies, will be addressed. I will present evidence that as we became human, a new form of collective life began to emanate, not just from groups, but from the very associations of which all groups are comprised—a life force in possession of such power that, with time, the laws of human nature would harness the natural laws of the earth.

---

[18]This is how I first began to conceive of the mentally ill as martyrs to our humanity.

CHAPTER 6

THE SACRED DISEASE
and
THE ORIGIN OF BELIEVING

A different drummer

Many years ago, while stopped at a traffic light, I saw a woman walking along a crowded street completely absorbed in a lively conversation with herself, replete with vigorous gesticulations and body posturing to emphasize each verbal interchange. Did this person have schizophrenia? No, I thought. She was too appropriately dressed, too aware of navigating through the foot traffic, and although it struck me as out of place, the conversation seemed plausible. Mental illness is often diagnosed by identifying the intensity of emotion along a geometrically upward sloping curve. It is only when the curve starts heading almost straight upward, denoting orders of magnitude greater emotional intensity, that the condition warrants a diagnosis as a sickness. My final diagnosis: she was talking on a cell phone headset.

Common words take on different and specific meanings when adopted by medicine. The word that has been sifted down through the attempts of generations of doctors to land on a term describing the behavior and affect manifested in schizophrenia is *bizarre*. I now find this term offensive, reeking of ignorance, and contributing to the stigma of this condition. A key indication in the diagnosis of schizophrenia is a disconnected quality about patients' behavior resulting from the fact that their emotional contact with the social environment is disrupted by the hyperactive thought process inside their minds. As they walk down the street, they are truly marching to a different drummer.

Had the cell phone woman been living with schizophrenia, her gestures would be more staccato and intense. Perhaps her dress might not conform to fashion. Her stride would not be attuned to the flow of movement around her, with generally decreased modulation in response to other people. Admittedly, this could describe a large segment of the population, but to the trained eye, there is a magnitude of intensity that, in its totality, is distinguishable from the mere oddness of normality.

The concept of intentionality, the direction of a motivation as discussed previously, is important in understanding schizophrenia. Normally, emotions are felt to be derived from oneself, perhaps an emotional response to some external event; and then one forms an intention, and the emotion is transformed into motivation. Gavin de Becker in *The Gift of Fear: Survival Signals that Protect Us from Violence,* (1997) stresses the importance of believing in the accuracy of one's fear as a signal of real danger. When you feel someone else's threatening intentions toward you, you need to set in motion your own intentions toward that person.

A paradox previously mentioned with respect to melancholia takes a different twist in schizophrenia. In melancholia, the patient appears from the outside to be trapped inside his mind, but from the inside, the patient perceives himself as painfully embedded in an intensely social experience. For people afflicted with schizophrenia, although much of their lives are lived inside their minds, both they themselves as well as outside observers perceive them to be responding to intentions that arise outside their mind.

A classic presentation of schizophrenia is a young person expressing the conviction that the metal braces on her teeth are picking up radio waves transmitted as thoughts directly into the patient's mind. That kind of symptom is specifically indicative of schizophrenia, and there is virtually no other illness that could produce it (except for some exceedingly rare neurological conditions). I concluded that the experience of one's thoughts emanating from an external source is the most essential feature of schizophrenia. This concept goes beyond the idea of paranoia, because the schizophrenic experience spans the full spectrum of emotion, not just fear and anger. A patient with schizophrenia is enthralled in thoughts determined by an intentionality whose transparent source, to both the patient and observer alike, is external to the patient.

The onset of schizophrenia can be rapid. Among the most troubling moments in my career were instances of early recognition of the unmistakable symptoms of this dreaded scourge in young adults. A bright young man sat in my office for the first time describing how, on the way home from college, he became convinced that license plates on the cars around him contained encrypted messages sent from a mysterious intelligence meant for him alone. It was the hesitancy with which he disclosed these experiences to me, as if he was not sure I could be trusted with information of such cosmic significance, that gave me the sinking feeling his life would henceforth be blighted by a sickness as cruel as it is mysterious. Unfortunately, my fears proved all too correct.

Insanity

During my wife Ann's rising career in the administration of the University of Maryland, I was in the position of being the chatty spouse of an increasingly important player in the state politics that are part of a large public university. Inevitably, in social interactions I could not avoid admitting that, yes, I am a psychiatrist. There is a curious paradox in people's responses to this disclosure. One common rejoinder is, "Oh, we're all a little crazy, aren't we?" Presumably, this reaction relates to the fact that anxiety and depression are accepted as normal, everyday emotions. However, there is also a hint of skepticism in the comment that mental illness exists at all, arising from a suspicion that patients only want attention and perhaps should be told to suck it up and live with it like the rest of us.

Then there is the opposite reaction, which cuts to the purpose of the essay: fear. Since I am thought to be in regular contact with crazy people, some people I meet actually flinch as if to protect themselves from mysterious contagions or, even more commonly, will assume I have the power to detect some depravity that lurks inside the recesses of their own minds. Occasionally, I was moved to reassure some folks who seemed genuinely concerned as to their own mental health.

If you ever visit Colonial Williamsburg, be sure not to miss the "Public Hospital for Persons of Insane and Disordered Minds" to get an idea of what counted as enlightened treatment of the mentally ill at the time of the Revolution. Note the iron rings on the walls of the rooms to which the patients were chained. We mental health professionals proudly picture *Pinel at the Salpêtrière*, the painting by Tony Robert-Fleury of Frenchman Philippe Pinel (1745-1826), considered the first modern psychiatrist, as he orders shackles removed from the insane in a Paris asylum in 1795. For the most part, the history of stigma arises from fear inspired by schizophrenia, which afflicts nearly one percent of the world's population across virtually all cultures and environments.

By far the most important breakthrough in the treatment of schizophrenia occurred in May 1952 when two French psychiatrists, Pierre Deniker and Jean Delay, published a study of a surgical anesthetic given to patients at the psychiatric Hôpital Sainte-Anne in Paris. The drug was chlorpromazine, later marketed as Thorazine. The results were dramatic. Without inducing excessive sedation at moderate doses, the drug brought about immediate improvements in the patients' emotions and behavior. It acted by blocking the neurotransmitter dopamine in the brain; all subsequent antipsychotic medications have retained this mechanism at their core.

Prior to Thorazine, the main drugs available for treating schizophrenia were barbiturates, which merely sedated patients without affecting their psychosis. The vivid experience of delusions (false beliefs) and hallucinations (false perceptions, mostly hearing voices) persisted. When I rotated through psychiatry in medical school in the 1960s, we were still taught how to wrap a patient into a *wet pack*, which from time immemorial had been the established treatment for intractable agitation. A sheet folded diagonally to form a long ribbon about two feet in width and soaked in cold water was firmly wound around the patient to immobilize the arms and legs, like a mummy. As the sheet warmed up from the patient's body heat, the patient would be calmed and fall into an exhausted sleep.[19]

Later, I would wonder how many times it had been performed on my aunt.

Kathryn

As a boy, I spent the summers with my grandmother in her rambling house in Quogue on the south shore at the east end of Long Island. There were no major roads out to the East End, and from the City, it seemed like an all-day drive past acres and acres of farms with vast flocks of white ducks and sprawling potato fields and through countless small villages. My grandmother presided over our far-flung family in the summer, and every morning, I would bicycle into town to pick up the newspaper for her and then spend time talking with her while she had breakfast on a tray in bed. She would let me have a piece of her melba toast and drink the last dregs of her coffee, which I thought were delicious.

An elegant Southern sadness surrounded my grandmother. The largest picture on her desk was of a beautiful young woman with long dark hair. One day I asked

---

[19] If you are an insomniac, try getting very cold and then warming back up again.

who this person was, and I clearly remember her response. She told me that the woman in the picture was her daughter Kathryn, my father's younger sister. Kathryn always wanted to be an actress and had joined a theater group that studied a "new kind of acting from Russia" in which she was trained to "become" the person she was portraying. She told me that it made Kathryn sick. "She got lost in the character she tried to become and never found her way back to herself," she said. My aunt had presumably been involved in method acting, founded by Konstantin Stanislavski. I assumed she had died of this mysterious condition, and in the way that children do, simply accepted it as something that sometimes happens to people.

Over the years, a rumor quietly spread among my generation of cousins that the beautiful woman in the picture was still alive, living in a sanatorium somewhere. Her fate was somehow maintained as something peripheral to our lives and a circumstance best left undiscussed.

However, after I became a psychiatrist, my father told me that Kathryn was floridly psychotic as a young woman and remained actively delusional her entire life. She had severe schizophrenia. This was long before any medications were available, and she, like most people with schizophrenia in those days, spent her life in a mental institution, where my father, unbeknownst to us, visited her regularly. He told me she would sometimes talk "repetitive nonsense" during his visits, and sometimes be withdrawn.

As my father's health declined, he became increasingly alarmed at what would happen to his chronically ill sister. Because I was now the active physician in the family, he asked me to visit her and assess her circumstances. I flew up to a state mental hospital north of New York City and, accompanied by a cousin, met our aunt at last. She was in a small, stark room, crumpled into a fetal position with a feeding tube in her stomach and an IV in her arm. We spent an hour with her, during which time we both determined that she was comatose and were told by the staff that she had been in this state for many years.

She died several months later. It was with Kathryn's body lying before me in a small room in the funeral home that I began to reflect on her life and illness. At the hospital, all my attention had been absorbed by searching for any small sign of consciousness. Of course, I knew many patients with chronic schizophrenia, and I was often the only person who took an active interest in their inner lives.

People with treatment-resistant schizophrenia mostly live their lives within their heads, but they are active lives, at times full of drama and excitement as well as occasionally terror. As my aunt lay before me, I wondered what her inner life might have been. I pondered the reality that whatever it had consisted of was now gone without a trace.

Henceforth I was to think from time to time about those moments I spent with her in contemplation of the pathos of a wholly solitary inner life simply falling silent. Years later, I arrived at the conviction that the normal experience of thinking is not a solitary process. A central component of thinking—perhaps its very soul—springs from a communal source that, however isolated the thinker, reflects and connects each to everyone. And I realized that the vital connection to the social environment within which we all dwell is tragically disabled in schizophrenia.

Messages

In Hippocrates' day, epilepsy was known as the *sacred disease* because a convulsive episode, or seizure, gave the appearance that the patient had been violently seized by the gods. In the same way, schizophrenia might also have been thought of as a sacred disease because the patient's mind appears seized by the gods. Although occasionally patients with schizophrenia have delusions of God directly communicating with them, much more commonly, the intentional thought sources are from secular institutions, public personalities, or an assortment of anonymous people.

Once I consulted on a case in which a middle-aged man was withdrawn and in a constant state of anguish mixed with outrage that the FBI was continuously and precisely shooting "beams" directly at a specific small part of his anatomy. To me there was something ominous in his affect, and I was deeply impressed by the compassion of the physician who referred him and who employed him in his office. I was proud to have associations with such noble individuals. The virtues of compassion and commitment to confront the enemy of affliction with the weapon of knowledge and the wisdom of experience is the sublime ethos I so admired in my colleagues.

The suicide rate in schizophrenia is around 10 percent. I recall a single consultation with a young man midway through college. I was one of half a dozen psychiatrists with whom he consulted. About six months before, he had an initial episode of psychosis in which he experienced voices talking to him and paranoid delusions that his friends were conspiring against him. He received treatment with an antipsychotic medication—one of the many subsequent iterations of Thorazine—which controlled the hallucinations and delusions, but he was an intelligent young man and knew something in him remained profoundly altered. He was unusually insightful in putting his finger upon a central problem in schizophrenia. He could see that his friends, including his girlfriend, perceived his disability and backed away. I tried to explain that the symptoms of schizophrenia are frightening to people, but knew he was talking about a real aspect of his condition often not controlled by medication, and I chose not to refute it further.

For those who do not understand that the minds of patients with schizophrenia are enthralled elsewhere, there can be a disturbing eeriness, as those living with this perplexing condition seem not to be present to a degree. My interactions with these patients were among the most satisfying because, as I mentioned before, I was often the only person with whom they could talk freely about their inner lives. Upon getting acquainted with someone with chronic schizophrenia, as mentioned before, it becomes as inappropriate to identify them as "sufferers" as it is for people living with diabetes. They are living and dealing with their condition, which is to be greatly admired. Nevertheless, during my career, except for HIV before effective treatments, schizophrenia has been the most stigmatized of all illnesses, which causes isolation and loneliness.

I grew to admire the parents of these patients. My anger at the notion of the "schizophrenogenic mother," through a mixture of maternal overprotection and maternal rejection could cause schizophrenia has smoldered over the years. The parents of the patient who was to become my most effective teacher about the nature of schizophrenia were the most caring, elegant people imaginable. I followed this patient, my teacher, for thirty years and still correspond with her. She was one of my first patients when I started my practice, referred to me for an obsessive-compulsive problem. After that condition remitted, she went off to college. While she was in college, I received a call from her saying she had not slept for several weeks because "men were circling my apartment and wanted something from me." There it was. The cardinal symptom of schizophrenia: not just fearfulness, as one might feel when one is alone and imagining that something frightening might be happening, but a specific and vivid kind of experience that something *is* constantly happening, in this case that the people in the cars around her apartment possessed motivations that were singularly focused on her. What it was they wanted from her or intended to do was unclear. There was a detached quality to the fear in her voice, an enigmatic ambivalence in her response to the conviction that she was the intentional focus of all these individuals. Once you have heard the emotional timbre of schizophrenia a dozen times, it becomes unmistakable, perhaps because the ominous foreboding of what it heralds becomes indelibly associated with it.

Even with the benefit of every incremental improvement in the antipsychotic medicines that would periodically appear on the market, this patient (and many others) remained in a state of chronic psychosis. Generally, her delusions and hallucinations were exciting to her, with a constant jumble of disjointed experiences with pop singers and sundry former avant-garde musical figures unknown to me. She would proudly announce to me in the same sentence that she was married to Jack Kennedy and that she had written most of the Beatles' songs. While she was talking to me she would be continuously distracted by someone talking to her through the telephone hanging on my wall and then point out precisely where other voices were coming from around her head. She would also, in the same session, talk poignantly about the limitations in her life and realistically about her disability. She knew her delusions were part of her illness, but this did not have the slightest effect on the vivid experiences that continued to make up most of her life.

Perhaps the most important eureka moment in my study of the schizophrenia experience occurred during a seemingly trivial interaction with this patient. One day I asked her, "How do you drive with all these thoughts running through your mind all the time?" Her response was simple: "Dr. Wylie, don't you daydream while you are driving?" In that instant I began to understand the relationship between schizophrenia and normal thinking.

Believing in thinking

The severest mental illnesses are divided into (1) the anxiety disorders, which include panic disorder, phobic disorder, and obsessive-compulsive disorder; (2) the mood disorders, which include atypical depression, melancholic depression, and bipolar disorder; and (3) schizophrenia, standing alone is a thought disorder.

In 1911, the pioneering Swiss psychiatrist Eugen Bleuler (1950) established schizophrenia as a psychiatric (mind) disorder, not a form of early onset dementia (*dementia praecox*) as previously assumed. He coined the word *schizophrenia* because he thought the fundamental problem in this affliction was a splitting, or dissociation, between emotions and cognition. The thinking process is clearly awry in schizophrenia, but its felt experience is associated with intense emotion even though those afflicted may outwardly present with a *flattened* affect. Bleuler also made the distinction between *positive* (hyperactive) and *negative* (underactive) symptoms in schizophrenia.

As discussed, I gave a great deal of thought to the role of negative symptoms in depression and concluded they were either a secondary brain-shutdown response or a direct result of the inhibitory aspect of the hyperactive emotional process (anxiety) that is the heart of the experienced pathology. I followed along these same lines of thinking with respect to the negative symptoms of schizophrenia. In the aftermath of weeks of sustained and extremely agitated psychosis, a patient reported to me that he had "no thoughts at all," which was upsetting to him. The agitation of his raging hyperactive thinking had finally elicited a global shut-down response, which included the process of thinking itself, called *poverty of thought*, a symptom also seen in melancholia. This patient's experience would militate toward the brain-shut-down idea.

On the other hand, in the days before the widespread use of antipsychotic medications, it was not uncommon for patients to present in a catatonic state, frozen like statues, or to demonstrate *waxy flexibility* in which, although they were immobile, one could reposition their limbs as if they were mannequins. I view these states as manifestations of patients being locked into a *dynamic stasis*. Recall Andrew Solomon's description while depressed of thinking through the stages of walking to the bathroom but being unable to perform the action because he was paralyzed with fear. However, a person with catatonic schizophrenia could not convey such an experience, because the very thinking apparatus required to assemble such thoughts is exactly what is frozen solid in such a mental state.

I ended up at the same place as I had with depression regarding the significance of the negative symptoms in schizophrenia. I had observed evidence of both a reactive brain-shut-down response and, in catatonia, inhibition from the primary hyperactive pathology. Either way, patients with flattened affect would tell me about the emotional intensity of their inner experiences, which I viewed as the core of the problem. As in depression, for the purposes of my phenomenological inquiry, I could ignore the negative symptoms.

The most dramatic experience associated with schizophrenia is hearing voices, which I feel is a secondary response to the primary phenomenon of pathological hyperactivity in the thinking process. Hearing voices results from the intensity of the "incoming" thoughts somehow crudely enlisting the vocal apparatus associated with thinking to produce this phenomenon of *loud thoughts*, which are fragmentary and often layered with repetitive statements, such as, "You're bad" or "Do it." I consider these auditory hallucinations to be a secondary phenomenon because they are so rudimentary in their content compared to the elaborate prolixity of the thoughts experienced in schizophrenia. It is also the case that the nature and presence of hallucinations varies in different cultures (Bauer, 2011), while the core process of the thought disorder does not.

By the time my patient made that comment to me about daydreaming, I had accepted the conventional wisdom that abnormalities in the thinking process were the primary pathology in schizophrenia. But I had also long since decided that the phenomenology of all mental illnesses consists of hyperactivity generated by the loss of the regulation of normal *emotions*, analogous to cancer cells escaping from their normal regulation into unrestrained growth. But what possible emotions that functioned in the normal thinking process could lose their modulation to produce this illness?

Another symptom characteristic of schizophrenia is that the received thoughts jump around (*loose associations*) in a way that seems illogical to others but that makes utter sense to the patient. As well as a splitting between thought, emotions, and behavior, Bleuler felt the term *schizophrenia* applied to the fragmentation in these patients' thought processes. In the post-World War II psychoanalytic era, gurus abounded in the art of translating the psychological meaning of the psychotic productions of schizophrenia, called *primary process thinking*. Primary process thinking is similar to Freudian interpretations of dreams in which the powerful emotions involved in the id-superego dynamic determine the narrative instead of reality-based cognition. The core idea that schizophrenia represents intense emotions that overwhelm the thinking process is consistent with the following.

THE SACRED DISEASE 63

The principal aspect of schizophrenia so strange to the rest of us is that patients with schizophrenia continue to believe their thoughts are real. I had many conversations about the preposterous nature of the content of delusional thoughts that were going through their minds. I encouraged these patients to draw the distinction between acknowledging they were legitimately experiencing them and suspending their belief that they represented reality. I am convinced these patients believed me when I told them their thoughts were part of their illness; nevertheless, that knowledge did not penetrate their much stronger belief that the content of their thoughts was real. These observations caused me to think deeply about the phenomenon of belief. What does it mean to have a "strong" belief? Obviously the strength of the belief in the case of schizophrenia has nothing to do with how real the object of the belief is. These delusions do not have any premise other than the subjective reality that they are ardently experienced by the patient to be thoughts of external beings who intensely and intentionally communicate to them.

Spurred by my conviction that the intentionality of the emotional experience in melancholia emanates from the social sphere, I began to think schizophrenia must involve a similar pathological process but played out in the realm of thought. In early hominins, mental attachment to the group must have elicited strong emotions in them, much as they do today. In other words, there was probably a strong bond formed around the moment-by-moment collective experience of belief. Perhaps we can think of this bond as similar to the belief in a set of political or religious tenets that bind together the believers. Is not belief the emotion that motivates allegiance and loyalty?

Rooting for the Yanks?

I began to consider the possibility that normal thinking involves communication with the belief systems from the various groups with which we identify ourselves. These systems do not exist as logical trains of thought but consist of firm emotional attachments to certain values (*rules*) associated with social groups; the simultaneous and intensive experience of receiving these social cues might explain the illogical loose associations characteristic of schizophrenic thinking. For example, the psychologist Jonathan Haidt, in his book *The Righteous Mind: Why Good People Are Divided by Politics and Religion* (2012), offers evidence that the differences between conservatives and liberals involve the dissimilar emphasis each group places in six belief categories: important issues to liberals are care/harm, liberty/oppression, and fairness/cheating, whereas for conservatives the most important issues are loyalty/betrayal, authority/subversion, and sanctity/degradation. A more general difference might be belief in the individual and hierarchy by conservatives versus the collective and equality by liberals. In the thinking process, one is in constant communication with various nested groups (via watching a favorite cable news channel, for example). We remain unaware of believing in a particular value system because we are unconsciously immersed within our beliefs in the same way that fish swim together in water.

In the thought-provoking book *Far from the Tree: Parents, Children, and the Search for Identity* (2012), about parents and their exceptional children, author Andrew Solomon writes, "The rich culture of Deafness, the LPA [Little People of America]-centered empowerment of dwarfism, ... the self-actualization of the autism rights brigade—none of this is really present in the world of schizophrenia." Perhaps the reason for this lack of group identity is that in schizophrenia, the very means by which group identities are formed is itself disrupted. But what is the nature of that disruption?

Certainly there has been a great deal of emotion associated with group membership throughout recorded history—for example, from differing religious sects and opposed political parties to warring nations—and there is evidence that our species was involved in intergroup violence in prehistoric times (Keeley, 1996). Could it be that the emotion generated by the competition between groups becomes disordered in schizophrenia?

In fact, the term "belief" originally referred exclusively to one's loyalty and affinity, such as when people say that they believe in a sports team, which clearly carries an emotional and competitive connotation. William Cantwell Smith points out in his *Belief and History* (1977) that it has only been since the Enlightenment era, when knowledge became more theoretical, that the word *belief* started to be used in reference to accepting a theoretical proposition, such as natural selection, on the basis of scientific evidence. Now with our divided politics, we are witnessing a reversion to its original meaning.

The origin of believing

At one point in my contemplation of this condition I wondered if the emotion in schizophrenia represented exactly this competitive-loyalty component so prominent in group alliances of modern humans. Was the emotion that breaks down in schizophrenia akin to, say, the cheering and booing at Yankee Stadium?

Indeed, competitive sentiments of group loyalty are not only manifest in chimpanzee behavior, but also, as I will eventually discuss, probably have actively evolved during our own species' evolution (Bowles, 2009). However, in my conversations with patients with schizophrenia, I could not perceive any emotions remotely related to group competition or loyalty. Certainly there are disjointed thought-messages from external agents, which sometimes are hostile to the patient, but these are private communications, and violence is always reactive. The nature of the intense emotions elicited reminded me more of the dominance–submission relationships I had observed in prison.

For example, in the Washington D.C. Navy Yard shootings in 2013, initially people assumed that the perpetrator was a terrorist motivated by hostile group beliefs. It turned out he was living with schizophrenia. In an email recovered by the FBI, he expressed his motive: "Ultra-low frequency [microwave] attack is what I've been subject[ed] to for the last 3 months, and to be perfectly honest that is what has driven me to this." The emotional mechanism itself whereby the authority of groups normally communicates with their obedient members reverts in schizophrenia into an intense dominance–submission relationship. It is the process of believing that is awry.

As I settled into the idea that schizophrenia is a disturbance in the communication from one's groups, I decided that the act of believing is *motivated by a felt emotion derived from the primate feeling of submission*. My inclination was to cast my mind back through deep time and consider how this facet of our communication evolved. I considered that the principal function of group identities in modern times is to bind together large groups, e.g.: countries, religions, ethnic groups, in competition with each other. However, after pondering the evolutionary meaning of schizophrenia, I concluded that this binding-through-competition function must have been a recent adaptation resulting from unique evolutionary developments in our own species, which I will address in Chapter 9, "Modern Humans: The Enigma of Vanity."

The function of binding large groups through members' feelings of loyalty must have been derived from a far more ancient phenomenon that existed within the small groups of pre modern hominins who spent their entire lives with the same relatively small group of people and had no need for modern mass group identities. Within these small groups the emotion of believing surely was fundamental to communication.

Because schizophrenia is such a crippling, evenly distributed, and widespread disorder, and because it leaves spoken language ability largely intact, I began to think the aspect of communication function that it disabled, which operates in the background, is a vestige of something far more central to prior species of hominins. In other words, this one facet of modern communication that serves to transmit group beliefs and competitive loyalty had been the only form of language communication at one time and therefore essential to hominin survival.

What if, prior to modern humans and our complex, multifaceted vocal language, communication was solely motivated by obedience to the evolved authority of groups? The goal of communication for the members of a group would have been to ascertain from one another how together they should coordinate behavior in such a way as to maximally benefit the group as a whole. This would be analogous to a group of believers discussing how to behave in a manner consistent with their shared beliefs. It is likely that this ancient component of our modern language, which has receded into the background of our communication, is disabled in schizophrenia.

Group selection

For the entire forty years that my wife, Ann, has worked at the University of Maryland, I attended only a handful of lectures there. I heard John Nash give a talk on economics, mostly out of my interest in listening to someone who apparently completely recovered from severe schizophrenia only to see his son develop it. I was certainly not going to miss a lecture by my hero, E. O. Wilson, on November 12, 2008, to celebrate (three months early) the bicentennial of the birth of Charles Darwin on February 11, 1809 (the day before Abraham Lincoln's). At one point, someone in the audience asked whether there was still room for the butterfly net in entomology. Without missing a beat, he said, "You betcha," imitating Sarah Palin's famous debate comeback, the 2008 presidential election having occurred the week before. Wilson is a wonderfully charming Southern gentleman with a twinkle in his eye, and I admire him enormously.

I was doubly interested because some months earlier I had read with surprise and delight an article that he co-authored with David Sloan Wilson (no relation) roundly endorsing the idea of group selection in the *Quarterly Review of Biology* (December, 2007). E. O. Wilson's validation of group selection brought perhaps the most controversial of all of Darwin's ideas out of the shadows and made it respectable again almost overnight.

I became familiar with Darwin's concept of group selection in my prison days when first reading through his great treatises. In contemplating the problem of why humans are cooperative in the face of the dog-eat-dog, survival-of-the-fittest world he was discovering (and creating), Darwin struck on the idea of group selection:

> There can be no doubt that a tribe including many members who, from possessing in a high degree the spirit of patriotism, fidelity, obedience, courage, and sympathy, were always ready to give aid to each other and to sacrifice themselves for the common good, would be victorious over most other tribes; and this would be natural selection (Descent of Man, 1871, p. 166).

This one short paragraph, even though not widely remarked upon, has had nearly as much popular influence as the idea of natural selection. The reason for its power is that the unassuming paragraph flows so naturally from the underlying assumption of Darwin's main theory of evolution.[20] He struck on his idea of natural selection when he read Thomas Malthus' calculations that life is an endless struggle for scarce resources; if resources increase for some reason, the population will also increase until there is scarcity again. Darwin simply applied this endless struggle for scarce resources paradigm to groups. So human hyper-cooperation is the legacy of a long succession of victories between chronically warring tribes, which he claimed could be a form of natural selection. This is a powerful idea.

The virtues from group selection that Darwin puts first are basically hierarchical military virtues associated with the political right: "patriotism, fidelity, obedience, [and] courage." Then, as if behind the battlefront, the more empathetic, collective

---

[20] Darwin's other assumption was drawn from his friend, Charles Lyell that existing geology is the result of small effects over vast periods of time.

values may secondarily percolate up (associated with the political left): "sympathy . . . always ready to give aid to each other and to sacrifice themselves for the common good." The bottom line is that our virtue is a result of chronic war.

Following along this logic, the Nazis claimed to inherit the genetic stock of the warlike Germanic peoples who, as a result, had evolved superior virtues; so in the post-war period, the idea of group selection in academia became tainted. However, the evolutionary gorilla in the academic living room was the superior capacity of humans for productive cooperation compared to its rudimentary presence in apes; how could this be explained without invoking some form of group selection?

In 1964, British biologist William Hamilton demonstrated that insects could be altruistic in proportion to their family relatedness. Fueled by the popularity of Richard Dawkins' *The Selfish Gene* (1976), leaping from insect to human behavior, *kin selection*—basically nepotism—was enthusiastically embraced as a large part of the explanation for human cooperation. In kin selection, identical genes are endowed with the capacity to recognize and cooperate with one another in blood relatives. Because a given gene is nothing more than information, it does not matter which version gets into the next generation; so family members evolve to help each other get at least one version of their common genes into the next generation.

In 1971, biologist Robert Trivers spelled out the evolutionary logic of *reciprocal altruism*: within relatively small, stable groups in which everyone has a sense of how reliable everyone else is, it is a winning strategy to help people who help you. Since then, kin selection and reciprocal altruism have been accepted as the default explanation for why humans are so much more cooperative than other primates. Translated into the language of the political right, family ties and transactional business relationships have made us cooperative.

In this context, the E.O. Wilson and D.S. Wilson article, "Rethinking the Theoretical Foundation of Sociobiology" (2007) was, and still is, viewed as heretical:

> The problem is that for a social group to function as an adaptive unit, its members must do things for each other. Yet, these group-advantageous behaviors seldom maximize relative fitness within the social group. The solution, according to Darwin, is that natural selection takes place at more than one level of the biological hierarchy. Selfish individuals might outcompete altruists within groups, but internally altruistic groups outcompete selfish

groups. This is the essential logic of what has become known as multilevel selection theory.

In a section entitled "Individuals as Groups," the two Wilsons point out that group selection obviously had played a role in assembling cells into individuals and even in assembling eukaryotic cells from precursor prokaryotic ones like bacteria. They assert that the high level of cooperation in *eusocial* insects like ants—E. O. Wilson's field of study—was the result of group selection and assume that group selection played a large role in human evolution[21] while suggesting that much of it happened recently due to the influence of culture. They end the paper on a humorous note:

> When Rabbi Hillel was asked to explain the Torah in the time that he could stand on one foot, he famously replied, "Do not do unto others that which is repugnant to you. Everything else is commentary." Darwin's original insight and the developments reviewed in this article enable us to offer the following one-foot summary of sociobiology's new theoretical foundation: "Selfishness beats altruism within groups. Altruistic groups beat selfish groups. Everything else is commentary."

From the moment I first read Darwin's description of group selection, I grasped its power to explain the association between cooperative loyalty and a competitive us-vs.-them mentality. But my patients with schizophrenia were telling me something different—that competitive loyalty, and ultimately war, is not the deepest source of human cooperation. Indeed, as will be discussed in Chapter 8, it stretches credulity to attribute to chronic war the cooperation required for our forebear species to colonize the vast continent of Eurasia. They had enough going on as it was—like sharing caves with giant hyenas in China (Boaz and Ciochon, 2004).

---

[21] E. O. Wilson finally unfurled his own new theory of human evolution in 2012 in *The Social Conquest of Earth*. He has now determined that group selection in eusocial insects resulted from building nests, and he speculates that it occurred in hominins when they controlled fire, because they thereafter stayed together in camps that needed defending. A point of agreement is that we both think that a change in social organization caused a shift to group selection in hominins.

Relational genes

My observations of melancholia prepared me to interpret schizophrenia as evidence that in hominins, social emotions and motivations had greatly strengthened and consolidated into a symbiotic relationship with individuals with whom they evolved to be in constant communication. Presumably then, as now, this communication involved group norms and rules for the benefit of the group, in order to counteract *decisively* the anti-social impulses of individuals. But had this communication from groups revealed by schizophrenia evolved by means of group selection?

The assumption made by both Darwin and the Wilsons is that the fundamental unit upon which group selection rests is the kinship group, the family tribe. So the whole theory of group selection also rests on kin selection and family ties—and that is where I part company with the concept. It is simply not believable to me that the entire edifice of human associations that has catapulted us into who we are today rests on genes recognizing themselves in families.

In an ironic turn of thought, while reading Richard Dawkins' *The Selfish Gene* (1976), the idea that genes (as opposed to individuals) could be the source of evolved (altruistic) intentions opened my mind to the possibility that the phenomenon of group authority-and-obedience could be the product of *relational genes*. Instead of group selection occurring top-down from unwieldy family groups, why wouldn't it make more sense that group selection occurs bottom-up from natural selection of relationship permutations whether within or between frequently interacting groups. Since the basic unit of selection is a group of only two, this process should be called *relational selection*. Relationships would be competing to survive and reproduce, as opposed to individuals doing so.

The major point to note is that the fitness of relationships would be determined largely by their retrospective *productivity and fecundity* and not their ability to win a continuous Malthusian struggle with one another. The crucial point of departure is that this is natural selection not of the fittest individual, but the most productive relationship, and *that* would be group selection. **My proposal here is that human evolution occurred when the benefits of association began to eclipse those of individual fitness.**

So when my patient with schizophrenia compared her inner life to daydreaming, my mind immediately flashed to the reality that a substantial source of our normal thinking emanates from this relational and shared *group space*, which consists of norms and values to which we passionately submit. Belief is the feeling of freely submitting (obedience) to group authority. My proposal is that the human family arose as a result of the individual dominance and submission mentalities merging into the single collective entity of authority, while evolving language with the ability to communicate to and among the individual (obedient) members of groups.

Then it would be regulation of the communication function of group authority that becomes unhinged by feedback reverberation in schizophrenia, exposing, by virtue of its intensity, the dynamic of its inner thought language. People with schizophrenia lack the ability to form identities because the very mental apparatus whereby groups communicate with individuals is disabled.

I realized that the feeling of believing mediates our obedience to authoritative codes within the nested groups in which we all live, immersed together as if creatures in the sea. At the moment of my patient's comment about waking dreams while driving, I conceived the source (or intentionality) of the authority that had commanded this same believing in our ancestral species. The intentional source of the process of believing had been like an ageless captain at the helm of the vessel that had borne our distant ancestors in their voyage through the eons. Schizophrenia exists as an emotional fossil of the most central animating experience for all who took that voyage; which is to say, everyone.

In the next two chapters, the subject shifts from psychiatry to human evolution and the science of paleoanthropology. In this second segment, I utilize the emotional fossils found in mental illness to tie together the facts of paleoanthropology and infer a causal evolutionary narrative of our inner mental life. I will propose a cascade of evolutionary events that could have rendered apes into a new form of life. Prior to the evolution of our own species, intentions of hominin *individuals to survive* were subsumed into collective intentions arising from the ascendance of natural selection for the decisive benefits of *coordinating their behavior*.

Please continue to keep in mind the essay's clinical goal to associate the experience of mental illness with the universal legacy of our evolutionary past.

PART TWO

MIND MEETS MATTER

CHAPTER 7

A NEW FORM OF LIFE

Stories

The most gripping aspect of Charles Darwin's and Alfred Russel Wallace's discovery of natural selection is that it proved humanity's creation to be a truly epic saga. Science remains in the early stages of revealing what are only fragmentary glimpses of this journey.

I propose that human nature evolved in response to three successive reconfigurations of social structure, with the most ancient being hierarchy. Adaptations to living in a hierarchical social ecology include our capacity for politics, which is the ability to compete strategically for dominance.

From studying the disorders of depression, I recognized that fears of separation and social entrapment are central to binding groups together. From studying schizophrenia, I was led to envision a unique mode of communication directed from the hominid group-organism to its individual constituents. Then there is the manic phase of bipolar disorder. However, because mania pertains only to we newly arrived *Homo sapiens*, it does not make an early entrance onto the stage.

The climax of this drama is the decisive moment six million years ago that launched our hominin tribe. My view is that a unique evolutionary transformation became the seed that would with time blossom into the being that inspired Hamlet to exclaim, "What a piece of work is man!"[22]

---

[22] The irony in Hamlet's monologue will emerge in Chapter 9, "Modern Humans: The Enigma of Vanity."

The beginning

The earth came into being violently 4.6 billion years ago when cosmic debris of increasing sizes imploded with accelerating force. Then about a billion years later, life appeared. There are biological forces that keep living things apart and those that bring them together. The most significant milestones in the history of life involved processes that drew single organisms together to coordinate their functions, thereby creating more complex organisms. About a half billion years ago, solitary cells engaged in just such a process resulting in all subsequent species of multicellular organisms (the Cambrian explosion). The rudimentary *intent* of a single cell to survive was forfeited to become one small part of a collective intent for many cells to survive. Whereas that cell had been out in the world all alone, it was now surrounded in productive harmony with others.

Could a final repetition of this drama be the human narrative?

Although our tribe suddenly coalesced six million years ago, the first steps in the human journey occurred 52 million years ago when primates began cohering into groups. Susanne Shultz and her colleagues at the University of Manchester (2011) hypothesized that group formation may have begun when primates shifted away from a nocturnal existence into functioning by day, when they were more vulnerable to predation. There are certainly more eyes to look out for danger in a group, but why issue a danger warning if I am safe at a distance? In the formation of groups, from the point of view of the individual, there is always a trade-off between looking out for number one and accruing the protective benefits of living in a group.

The usual paradigm is to conceive the evolution of groups from the point of view of natural selection exclusively occurring at the level of the individual (or gene). In this narrative, the paradigm shifts from the point of view of individuals to that of groups, starting from their very inception in our Order Primates. A helpful perspective in understanding the nature of group selection is to think about the first group-selected gene. A group-selected gene confers no advantages without a group. It takes two to tango. It is only when two individuals contribute *complimentary* components of a relational gene conferring advantages to the couple that group selection commences and expands from the ground up. But where is the expression (phenotype) of that first gene to be found?

Indeed, where is any group to be found, and what exactly is it?

What and where is a group?

The concept of a phenotype lies at the heart of what is new in this interpretation of evolution through mental illness. Your genotype consists of all your genes that contain the coded *recipes* to synthesize your phenotype—you—the person reading this. We usually think of genes coding for physical characteristics like eye color and height, but this essay explores the reality that emotions and intentional motivations are also part of an inherited phenotype. Everyone knows that emotions are influenced by family and social environments during growth and development, but here we are concerned only with the inherited genetic portion subject to natural, group, and sexual selection.

The currently reigning paradigm of evolutionary psychology assumes the primacy of cognition over emotion-and-motivation: all groups are formed by individuals, each evolved to calculate strategically what benefits are contained in any cooperative interaction. But emotions need not play second fiddle to such cognitive calculations.

I propose that the social emotions described in the last four chapters exist within the relationships among the individuals of a group and are phenotypes of relational genes; a relational gene only becomes whole when its converse parts functionally fit together within a relationship. It is as if these genes within individuals code for musical instruments that are selected based on whether they harmonize with one another. Such genes evolve in each generation by first reconstituting themselves within a new network of relationships (phenotypes), the most productive permutations of which then are naturally selected *passively* at the end of each generation based on fecundity alone.

Life is the capacity to replicate and evolve. This living entity, the protagonist in this narrative, exists in the ethereal world of emotions that promote formation and survival of groups without regard to their physical environment. Far from being corrupted into tortured cognitive "Machiavellian" machinations (Byrne and Whitten, 1988), the emotions and motivations of groups possess a singular purity and constancy of purpose: that of ceaselessly pushing and pulling individuals together.

The villains in this drama in which the group is the hero are the antisocial contra-twins of fight and flight. I have introduced the protagonist emotions residing in primate groups as the two fundamental fears of interpersonal *separation* and of being *trapped* at the bottom or periphery of groups. Stated another way, the aversive motivation of these fears is elicited by increasing distances from attached personal relationships (for example, a pair-bond) and decreasing distances from the periphery of groups (as one approaches the dread of being *up against the edges* of a group). These two fears, one experienced as being pulled together and the other as pushed back in, exerted a relentless cohesive force that enters into a continuous dynamic with the primal responses of fight and flight. The result is that individuals were restrained from chasing one another out of their groups.

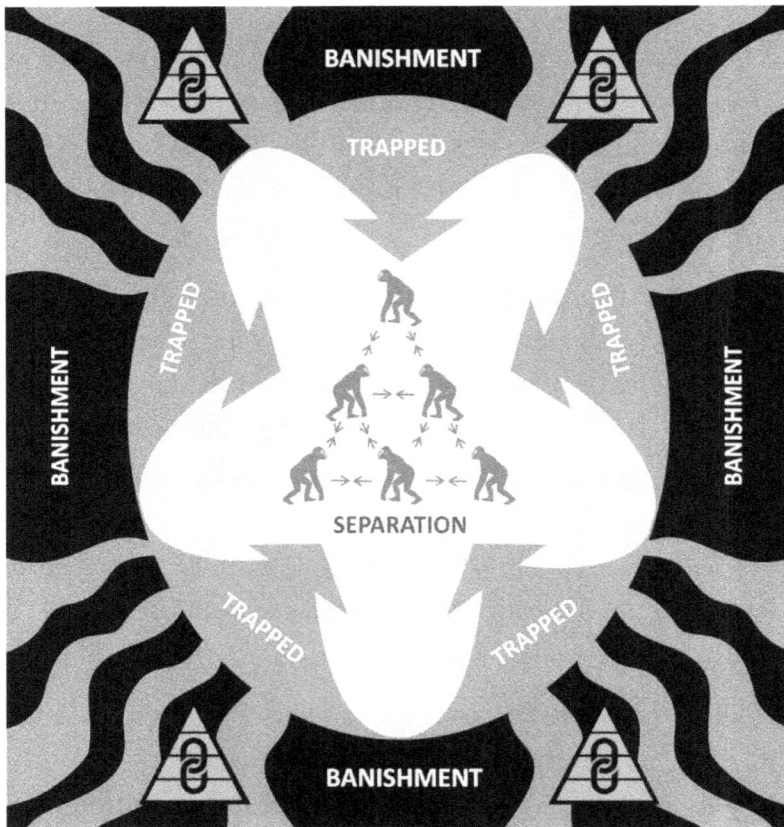

The rising internal stress caused by balanced interaction between these sets of opposing emotions and motivations—one from individuals and the other from the collective sphere—crystallized into the stable structure of nested pyramids. Hierarchies are comprised of the force of collective social emotions and motivations pressing inward from groups, locked into a dynamic stasis with the flesh and blood impulses of fight and flight pressing outward. The dominance and submissive mentalities are the alloyed precipitants of this dynamic stasis, which naturally self-organize into hierarchy.

The fundamental unit of behavior in a hierarchy consists of a political triangle: two attempting to *triangulate* (intimidate) a third. When the four possible political triangles between the same four individuals sort themselves out, the individual with the most alliances-through-intimidation ends up at the apex of a stable social pyramid in which three of the four members are "vertically" bound to the forth by bonds of dominance and submission. Within a group, all permutations of these triangles crystalize into the simple geometric form of nested pyramids. This hierarchical order reduces the level of disruptive behavior inside the system, and therefore enhances the collective security and survival of all the participants. A robust dynamic stasis is naturally obtained in which the fittest political practitioners dominate/intimidate those below at each nested level.

Just as birds became specialists in the spatial ecology of the air, primates became specialists in the emotional ecology of the dynamic hierarchies of their groups. Far from physical, this ecology is comprised of a fluid, publicly held registry of a group's most recent social interactions. In *Baboon Metaphysics: The Evolution of a Social Mind* (2007), authors Dorothy L. Cheney and Robert M. Seyfarth determined that every single baboon knows exactly where he or she stands at a particular moment in time, in their somewhat fluid hierarchies of about one hundred animals—and all behave according to the hierarchical rules of submitting to those dominant over you, and dominating those submissive under you.

A game is competition with rules. The fight and flight emotions were drawn into a game produced by their interaction with the two social fears of separation and entrapment. Over the course of millions of years, primates became the most intelligent animals on earth because they evolved competitive skills honed by playing this internal hierarchy game, which had become all-consuming, particularly among males. Once again, primate cognitions, focused on competitively reading each other's minds, are adaptations to an environment comprised entirely of social emotion.

It is fruitful to pause here and place the narrative within the context of one of the most hotly contested issues in the field of evolution. In 1972, Niles Eldredge and

Stephen Jay Gould published an often-cited essay, "Punctuated equilibria: An alternative to phyletic gradualism," in which they proposed that evolutionary change happened rapidly with long intervening periods of stability. In this same way, this narrative proposes three major reconfigurations that punctuate the evolution of social emotion—the one just discussed, beginning 52 million years ago with the formation primate hierarchies; then one initiated six million years ago when hominins split from apes; and one that arose with our own *Homo sapiens* species two to three-hundred-thousand-years ago.

Each of these changes happened with relative rapidity, and each created a new social environment, in response to which novel cognitions gradually elaborated as adaptations. So this model encompasses both punctuation and gradualism; three punctuated reconfigurations in emotion created three environments spawning gradual cognitive adaptations.

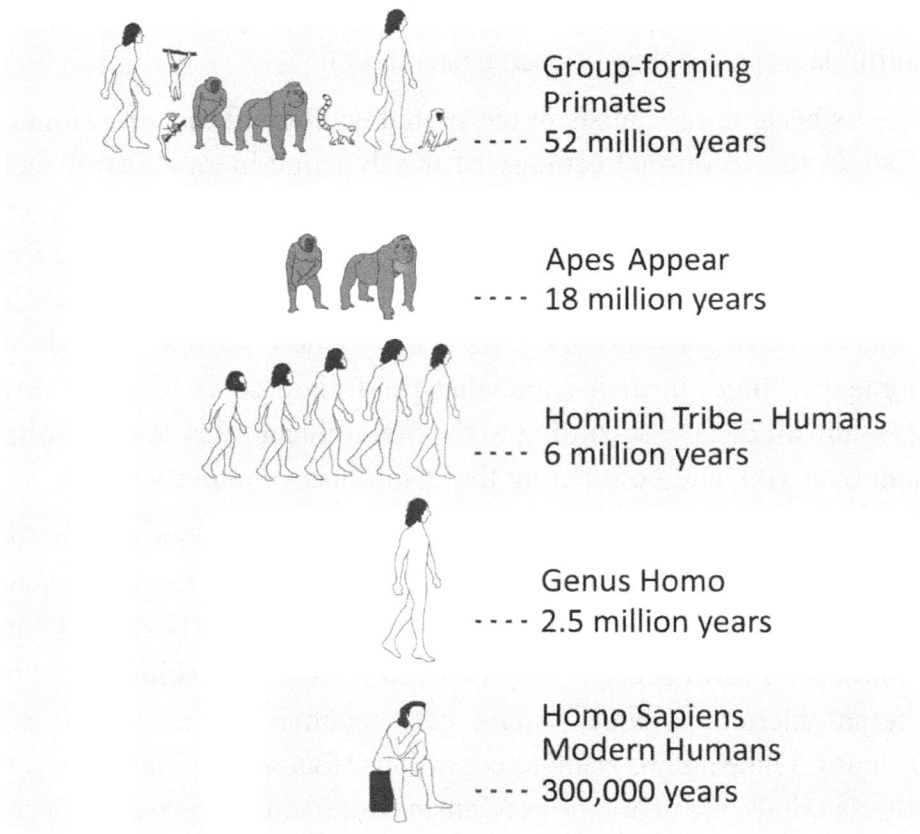

Group-forming
Primates
· · · · 52 million years

Apes Appear
· · · · 18 million years

Hominin Tribe - Humans
· · · · 6 million years

Genus Homo
· · · · 2.5 million years

Homo Sapiens
Modern Humans
· · · · 300,000 years

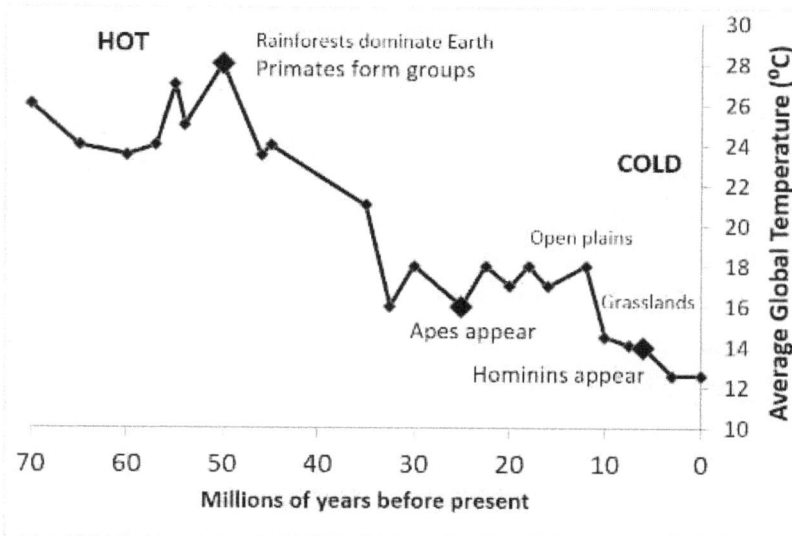

Approximately six million years ago, an environmental circumstance came to pass that I propose triggered a series of evolutionary events, one of which was unique in the history of life. Apes (large tailless primates) thrived in the forests of North Africa for millions of years before a precipitous five-million-year cooling period eventually drove apes into near extinction.

A genetic study using *Markovian coalescent analysis* demonstrates that chimpanzees underwent a dramatic population collapse around the time that hominins evolved (Prado-Martinez *et al.*, 2013). This important study calculates that, starting about six million years ago, the chimpanzee population dropped by a factor of 5 in the following four million years. The three ape "refuge" species left in Africa—gorillas, chimpanzees, and bonobos—hang on in isolated enclaves. The brutal fact of imminent extinction means the chimpanzee population was diminishing because too few young being born or if born, not surviving.

This is where our narrative begins to interpret the known facts and to posit a hypothetical mechanism for the human transformation. In this scenario, after 46 million years of primate social evolution, while the survival of individual chimps had become increasingly dependent on groups, their brains had evolved an addiction to their elaborate internal hierarchy game. But this day-to-day competition for rank was wasted energy, significantly constraining fertility and thus becoming a threat to their survival as a species. My proposal is that the unique hominin trajectory was launched by a cascade of simultaneous evolutionary events, the first of which produced the most efficient and fertile social system of all: monogamy.

Monogamy

E. O. Wilson, mentioned above, is a formidable philosopher of human nature. He bases his conclusions on his belief that cooperation in ants and other *eusocial* insects (bees, wasps, and termites) represents the closest animal model to human social cooperation. His main argument for the evolutionary narratives of eusocial insects and humans being identical is that, in terms of sheer biovolume, they and we are the most successful multi-celled creatures by far, and because nature is known to be both lazy and stingy, only one path could lead to such rare success.

In 2008, William Hughes, a British sociobiologist, took advantage of the rapidly advancing mathematical science of *ancestral state reconstruction* to determine that, despite sterile castes and queens in existing species, the original founding species of all eusocial insects were monogamous. This landmark study raised the possibility that although modern humans are not strictly monogamous (also with some queens), our original founding species might well have been.

Ever since a species of prairie vole was discovered to possess a high degree of monogamy, they have been the object of intensive research. Interest centers on the role in these rodents' monogamy of the neuropeptide *oxytocin*, which is also secreted in human mothers at childbirth and is thought to enhance bonding with their babies. In an article in *Science* (2015), Mariam Okhovat and her colleagues at the University of Texas found in a study conducted in the wild that higher rates of monogamy correlated with low population densities. They reasoned that if you are a male vole and are out foraging over long distances for too long a time (low density), the greater the chance that another male vole is having sexual contact with your own mate, making you a loser in the get-as-many-of-my-genes-as-possible-into-the-next-generation contest.

In other words, when the population is decreasing, as it was for apes when hominins arose, the wisest gene move is to stay put and keep an eye on a single female. Moreover, biological mathematician Sergey Gavrilets in 2012 modeled a shift from a mentality of sexual "appropriation" to one of pair-bond "production."

The anthropologist C. Owen Lovejoy in his seminal article, "The Origin of Man" (1981), stated: "The traditional view that early human evolution was a direct consequence of brain expansion and material culture is incorrect, and that the unique sexual and reproductive behavior of man [i.e.: cooperative monogamy] may be the *sine qua non* of human origin." His position was greatly strengthened by the discovery (published in 2009) of the 4.4-million-year-old hominin *Ardipithecus ramidus* fossils in which male canine teeth are much smaller than those of chimpanzees. Chimpanzees are highly competitive hierarchical apes (although bonobos are not so competitive) with a promiscuous mating system, and the smaller canines in "Ardi" could indicate a species with much reduced aggression. Dr. Lovejoy also thought small size differences between males and females in the Ardipithecus fossils indicate they were monogamous.[23]

Some monogamy facts: 85 to 95 percent of birds, 3 to 5 percent of mammals—but approximately 15 percent of mammals' primate component—are classed as monogamous (Díaz-Muñoz, 2013). Selected species of primates began evolving monogamous social systems about 16 million years ago, relatively late in their 52-million-year history of group living (Shultz, 2011). In each case, monogamy grew out of a promiscuous mating system (Opie, 2012), perhaps similar to that in chimpanzees or bonobos. Although paternal care can be a mating strategy for males in some promiscuous primate species (Smutts, 1992), genetic motivation (kin selection) for such care is absent because the paternity of offspring is most often unknown. In any event, it is likely that a transition from promiscuity to monogamy played a large role in hominin evolution, but with uncertainty as to how and when it occurred.

The front end: Sexual selection

The complete title of Charles Darwin's second great treatise is *The Descent of Man, and Selection in Relation to Sex* (1871). Interest generated by this book arose (and still arises) from the fact that Darwin was finally writing about our own species. But the second half of the title is what most intrigued me, particularly because he clearly felt that sexual selection was a major mechanism in human evolution. Darwin was not as interested in intra-sexual selection—males competing for access to females—as he was in intersexual selection, in which females select traits

---

[23] However under the sway of natural selection for the divided labor of teamwork, monogamous couples would evolve to differ in size in accordance with their differing functions.

in males that have no apparent survival value. His book describes these spectacularly curious male traits in birds in the precise, vivid language that is his hallmark:

> They charm the female by vocal or instrumental music of the most varied kinds. They are ornamented by all sorts of combs, wattles, protuberances, horns, air-distended sacs, top-knots, naked shafts, plumes and lengthened feathers gracefully springing from all parts of the body. The males sometimes pay their court by dancing, or by fantastic antics performed either on the ground or in the air (John Murray 2nd edition, page 359).

While thinking about how these male traits could have evolved by natural selection, Darwin, who famously suffered from psychosomatic symptoms, wrote to a colleague (1860) that "The sight of a feather of a peacock's tail, whenever I gaze on it, makes me sick." In what may be his most brilliant and courageous proposal, Darwin finally decided there was no other answer than that these female birds had developed a taste for beauty, which engendered pleasure, and that they themselves were doing the selecting without regard to natural selection.

In the following passage, Darwin appears to endow the quality of beauty with a Platonic reality to which the substance of the brain responds with pleasure. He then, in an afterthought, draws attention to the fact that, of course we modern humans also have developed "nearly the same" taste for beauty:

> With the great majority of animals... the taste for the beautiful is confined to the attractions of the opposite sex. The sweet strains poured forth by many male birds during the season of love are certainly admired by the females, of which fact evidence will hereafter be given. If female birds had been incapable of appreciating the beautiful colours, the ornaments, and voices of their male partners, all the labour and anxiety by the latter in displaying their charms before the females would have been thrown away; and this is impossible to admit. . . On the whole, birds appear to be the most aesthetic of all animals, excepting of course man, and they have nearly the same taste for the beautiful as we have. . . (p. 61).

This is definitely not the classical bottom-up natural selection of chance mutations in response to the environment. This is top-down selection conducted by the fully engaged mind of a living creature. Darwin also recognized that the female capacity to select male traits and the male traits themselves evolved in direct response to each other, a phenomenon called coevolution:

The male Argus Pheasant acquired his beauty gradually, through the preference of the females during many generations for the more highly ornamented males; the aesthetic capacity of females advanced through exercise or habit just as our own taste is gradually improved (p. 793).

In 1930, English polymath Ronald Aylmer Fisher updated Darwin's idea of co-evolution in sexual selection in his *The Genetical Theory of Natural Selection*. Darwin knew nothing about genes. But Fisher recognized the significance that offspring of the union between the peacock and the peahen, whether male or female, possessed both the genes for desiring fancy tails and the genes for the tails themselves. So in successive generations, selection for the genes of each are continuously linked together, as fancier tails spawned more refined tastes for even fancier tails. This creates a powerfully self-sustaining feedback loop that can rapidly spin off in its own internally willful direction without regard to the absence of any survival advantage. Fisher called this "runaway" evolution, and it is a strong candidate for punctuated evolutionary change. This process would only end when the peacock's tail becomes large enough to prevent survival before mating.

It seems natural that sexual selection was the evolutionary mechanism that drew the two sexes into a state of monogamous cooperation in response to the threat of extinction. Females with a feisty temperament, and an inclination to reject their more aggressive suitors, began to choose males who (1) were less dominant, (2) had higher levels of separation fear, (3) higher oxytocin, and (4) assisted in the care of offspring, started having more progeny that survived. Because of this evolved inclination arising in females, their successful male offspring became more and more disposed to stay with one female and assist with foraging for the family.

As part of a suite of adaptations for monogamy, females evolved to be continuously sexually receptive, rather than only during ovulation, which became concealed. The concealment of female fertility cycles most likely was adapted to allow for the *privatization* of sex that's essential for monogamy. Thus, along with increasing fear of separation, ongoing sexual contact became a powerful bonding agent in monogamy.

However, monogamous groups in nature are not particularly sociable due to concern about—you guessed it—infidelity. If you are a male and your wife bears someone else's children, as good a husband and father as you may be, biologically these good genes are not carried forward. So, for example, primate gibbons are monogamous, but they live in separate nuclear families having little to do with one another.

One way to look at the influence of social emotions is that they establish *rules*. The group's method of exerting its cohesive influence had for 46 million years been the establishment of the two transactional rules of a dominance hierarchy: feel/behave (1) submissive to dominant individuals and (2) dominant to submissive ones. When you think about it, the rules needed to live most productively in a closely bonded monogamous group comprise a good model for the rules of morality.

During my prison work, I first read Darwin's theory in *The Descent of Man* that in chronically warring groups, "an advancement in the standard of morality will certainly give an immense advantage to one tribe over another." Darwin was wedded to his core belief that natural selection always involved the element of Malthusian struggle for scarce resources, in this case between groups. Because the social structure in prison is made up of competing hierarchical (ethnic and racial) groups, it was an ideal environment to investigate the role of morality in this environment.

I saw a lot of loyalty in prison but not much morality. However, justice was a central issue there, not that anyone agreed about what it was in a given circumstance. Nevertheless, those convicts convinced me that they believed in justice, and it was they who started me on the road to propose that we are moral because we are just, and that *justice is a deeply evolved human instinct.* My simplistic thought back then was that the whole criminal justice system in which I was involved was only a modern iteration of an equivalent process that had gone on for millions of years in the groups of our hominin ancestors. Our morality is the legacy of our predecessors' relentless pursuit of justice through the millennia, but why did justice become the middleman between morality and its benefits, and what are the benefits of morality other than to win wars as Darwin had suggested?

I finally began to approach the answer to these crucial questions as I came to view melancholia as an emotional fossil. It was the rapid intensification of the fear of social entrapment-and-banishment that motivated morality by aversion: eight of the Ten Commandments mandate what should *not* be done. However, only when I learned from my patients that melancholic emotions and motivations possessed social intentionality directed at individuals did the inside story ⟨an indepe⟩ place. The conversion from the hierarchies of apes to the *organic* ⟨start f...⟩ e of hominins was mediated by a rapid intensification of melan- ⟨so⟩ into the intentionality of justice. In hominins, the socializing inten- ancholic fears galvanized into the collective dominance over individ- e recognize as *authority*—the authority of justice. I propose that this us transformation occurred with punctuated rapidity right at the begin- human evolution.

Upright posture is the earliest, most defining human trait and is evidence that the human transformation occurred "up front." Most consider that bipedalism evolved for one set of reasons (disappearing forests) and then *physically* led to later adaptations such as tool making and endurance running (Bramble and Lieberman, 2004). In the next chapter I propose the very different perspective that upright posture was intrinsic to a suite of simultaneous evolutionary events in the *mind* that thereafter remained the font of all subsequent human adaptations. Now I will discuss the Darwinian mechanisms behind a cascade of changes that rendered submission and dominance between ape individuals into obedience towards the authority of justice in hominin groups.

In the context of converting to monogamy under the threat of extinction, why could not a phenomenon exactly like sexual selection take place between the dominance and submission mentalities, transforming them into obedience and authority? A plausible first step could have been the following: pushed by increasing melancholic fears, female apes in a submissive mode could acquire a desire for males pursuing justice instead of dominance over their small sub-group. A shift in male motivation for dominance to that of justice would then evolve in response to the female motivation to select it. This female motivation would be not for the pleasure of beauty, as in the peahen, but for easing increased melancholic social fears. We love justice not because it makes us happy, but because it brings peace of mind. The genes for both dispensing and obeying justice would be passed down together within each of the male and female offspring of successive generations, and thus attain the same one-way-street effect as in sexual selection. The difference is that obedience to justice, once it enters the collective and relational realm, sheds all sexual affiliation.

work, hit upon the open-ended productivity of an organic social system. Those permutations of relationships that were not as productive as ones that were, failed to replicate successfully. Eons of striving for dominance inside the penitentiary of a hierarchy was finally harnessed by the collective impulse for justice, which as I have shown is the core of being human.

Dominance and submission cohabited within the mind of every primate creature for scores of millions of years—like an ancient couple whose marriage vows were consecrated on condition that they remain chaste: thereafter, whenever one awakened, the other was made to slumber. But now, the preordained moment had at long last arrived. It was time for dominance and submission to finally cleave together and consummate their hallowed union by pledging allegiance to a sacred covenant. Henceforth, those endowed with the will to dominate would solemnly pledge allegiance to justice, and those that had previously cowered as apes would proudly kneel in obedience to the authority of justice as humans. Welded together into an instrument of an ascendant being, they set forth to forge the new order of a just society.

The remarkable aspect of evolution by sexual selection is that it is driven by the desire for a trait, in this case the desire for justice. But as it proceeds, sexual selection becomes not only driven by the peahen's desire for the peacock's tail, but also by the peacock's desire to be desired for his tail. So what gave sexual selection the creative power to launch and then sustain our hominin tribe was, and still is, the additive effect of both the desire for justice and the desire to be just, both passed down together in successive generations tightly engaged in the pioneering of rightness and wrongness.

Under the protective shield of justice, groups of mated pair-bonds could evolve the productive benefits of coordinating and dividing the labor of childcare (Hrdy, 2006, Silk, 2007) and foraging for food. At the end of the day, those groupings of relationships that *believed* in the rules of this organic social structure would be naturally selected. The procreative benefits to individuals within a given group under this obedience–authority system would exceed any benefits of pursuing their own dominance.

The will to dominate in the ape mind transformed into the authority of justice in the early human mind by migrating from individuals to dwelling within the thin ether of relationships between individuals; no one could see it, but all could feel it. This invisible but biologically based will could be said to possess intentions, that is, a spirit—the human spirit. Human bonds animated by this still evolving spirit ultimately would become more powerful than those of blood, tribe, or country.

The larger picture is that 52 million years ago, fight and flight responses among primates were *compressed* by the collective social emotions into hierarchies comprised of the sustained mental states of submission and dominance. The narrative continues that, in a similar manner, these mentalities of submission and dominance were further compressed by social emotions into an organic structure consisting of obedience to collective authority motivated by guilt and shame on the part of individuals, and a collective rage for justice on the part of groups. No longer were primate individuals playing games according to the rules of a hierarchy; instead, the minds of hominin individuals became colonized and rendered obedient to the living evolving authority of their groups. Just as cells had formed into individual organisms hundreds of millions of years before, now individuals formed into organism-like groups that shared their mental and emotional life.

an independent social intentionality directed at individuals did the inside story start falling into place. The conversion from the hierarchies of apes to the *organic* social structure of hominins was mediated by a rapid intensification of melancholic fears into the intentionality of justice. In hominins, the socializing intentions of melancholic fears galvanized into the collective dominance over individuals that we recognize as *authority*—the authority of justice. I propose that this momentous transformation occurred with punctuated rapidity right at the beginning of human evolution.

Upright posture is the earliest, most defining human trait and is evidence that the human transformation occurred "up front." Most consider that bipedalism evolved for one set of reasons (disappearing forests) and then *physically* led to later adaptations such as tool making and endurance running (Bramble and Lieberman, 2004). In the next chapter I propose the very different perspective that upright posture was intrinsic to a suite of simultaneous evolutionary events in the *mind* that thereafter remained the font of all subsequent human adaptations. Now I will discuss the Darwinian mechanisms behind a cascade of changes that rendered submission and dominance between ape individuals into obedience towards the authority of justice in hominin groups.

In the context of converting to monogamy under the threat of extinction, why could not a phenomenon exactly like sexual selection take place between the dominance and submission mentalities, transforming them into obedience and authority? A plausible first step could have been the following: pushed by increasing melancholic fears, female apes in a submissive mode could acquire a desire for males pursuing justice instead of dominance over their small sub-group. A shift in male motivation for dominance to that of justice would then evolve in response to the female motivation to select it. This female motivation would be not for the pleasure of beauty, as in the peahen, but for easing increased melancholic social fears. We love justice not because it makes us happy, but because it brings peace of mind. The genes for both dispensing and obeying justice would be passed down together within each of the male and female offspring of successive generations, and thus attain the same one-way-street effect as in sexual selection. The difference is that obedience to justice, once it enters the collective and relational realm, sheds all sexual affiliation.

A plausible scenario is that a mechanism akin to sexual selection accomplished an initial rapid transformation from dominance to the authority of justice, and then subsequently this collective entity was sustained by natural selection. What force of natural selection was powerful enough to propel this evolutionary transformation from apes, and then sustain it for the millions of years of hominin evolution? The answer to this vital question comes from an unlikely source.

The back end: The natural selection of justice

Scots economist and moral philosopher Adam Smith is well known in his *Wealth of Nations* (1776) for attributing wealth to the division of labor, the self-interest of individuals being guided into productive engagement by an *invisible hand.* Smith is less known for his *Theory of Moral Sentiments* (1759), in which he singles out justice as the one moral sentiment indispensable to productive social functioning. A straightforward evolutionary interpretation of Smith's profound thinking is that the invisible hand is the naturally selected collective capacity to coordinate labor, and that *the coordination of divided labor is the principal hominin adaptation.*

Justice is the one virtue indispensable to productive social engagement because justice is the collective instinct naturally selected to allow the benefits of productive social engagement to take root and blossom.[24] We have prevailed not as individuals, but because we evolved the capacity to engage in ever more elaborate teamwork, and it has been the establishment of instincts for the rules of justice that permitted this organic social system to emerge and thrive. So here we have a more plausible evolutionary story for morality than the Darwinian-Wilsonian comrades-in-arms scenario.

The reason we find so many hominin fossils and none from apes during the early hominin era is not only because hominins lived in drier climates that preserved bones, but because their social structure promoted teamwork and was more successful from the beginning. Thus, hominins rapidly branched into many species and genera. By the happenstance of hard times, a founding species, with well-developed transactional intelligence and prehensile hands that could be put to

---

[24] Wolves coordinate hunting in packs and have been found to have the rudiments of justice (Bekoff and Pierce, 2009).

work, hit upon the open-ended productivity of an organic social system. Those permutations of relationships that were not as productive as ones that were, failed to replicate successfully. Eons of striving for dominance inside the penitentiary of a hierarchy was finally harnessed by the collective impulse for justice, which as I have shown is the core of being human.

Dominance and submission cohabited within the mind of every primate creature for scores of millions of years—like an ancient couple whose marriage vows were consecrated on condition that they remain chaste: thereafter, whenever one awakened, the other was made to slumber. But now, the preordained moment had at long last arrived. It was time for dominance and submission to finally cleave together and consummate their hallowed union by pledging allegiance to a sacred covenant. Henceforth, those endowed with the will to dominate would solemnly pledge allegiance to justice, and those that had previously cowered as apes would proudly kneel in obedience to the authority of justice as humans. Welded together into an instrument of an ascendant being, they set forth to forge the new order of a just society.

The remarkable aspect of evolution by sexual selection is that it is driven by the desire for a trait, in this case the desire for justice. But as it proceeds, sexual selection becomes not only driven by the peahen's desire for the peacock's tail, but also by the peacock's desire to be desired for his tail. So what gave sexual selection the creative power to launch and then sustain our hominin tribe was, and still is, the additive effect of both the desire for justice and the desire to be just, both passed down together in successive generations tightly engaged in the pioneering of rightness and wrongness.

Under the protective shield of justice, groups of mated pair-bonds could evolve the productive benefits of coordinating and dividing the labor of childcare (Hrdy, 2006, Silk, 2007) and foraging for food. At the end of the day, those groupings of relationships that *believed* in the rules of this organic social structure would be naturally selected. The procreative benefits to individuals within a given group under this obedience–authority system would exceed any benefits of pursuing their own dominance.

The will to dominate in the ape mind transformed into the authority of justice in the early human mind by migrating from individuals to dwelling within the thin ether of relationships between individuals; no one could see it, but all could feel it. This invisible but biologically based will could be said to possess intentions, that is, a spirit—the human spirit. Human bonds animated by this still evolving spirit ultimately would become more powerful than those of blood, tribe, or country.

The larger picture is that 52 million years ago, fight and flight responses among primates were *compressed* by the collective social emotions into hierarchies comprised of the sustained mental states of submission and dominance. The narrative continues that, in a similar manner, these mentalities of submission and dominance were further compressed by social emotions into an organic structure consisting of obedience to collective authority motivated by guilt and shame on the part of individuals, and a collective rage for justice on the part of groups. No longer were primate individuals playing games according to the rules of a hierarchy; instead, the minds of hominin individuals became colonized and rendered obedient to the living evolving authority of their groups. Just as cells had formed into individual organisms hundreds of millions of years before, now individuals formed into organism-like groups that shared their mental and emotional life.

For me, Tomasello is constrained by individual thinking; he finesses the cognitive Rubicon-that-must-be-crossed between perspective-taking and true collective intentionality by attributing the latter to the child's own "ability to self-regulate," which effectively strips intentionality from superego.[25] In my view, it is the reverse: the collective intentions of the superego (groups) have been naturally selected to *colonize* the child's mind for the benefits of teamwork. I propose that a collective intentionality has been broadly rooted in the relational ground of being human from the very beginning. However, these details pale next to Tomasello's achievement of providing compelling evidence in the crucible of science for that which is uniquely human within us.

In a summary passage, Tomasello places shared intentionality into its proper perspective:

> As a final attempt to characterize the monumental transformation of human ontogeny that shared intentionality has effected, let us invoke the grand evolutionary scheme of Maynard Smith and Szathmáry (1995). They identified eight major transitions in the evolution of complexity of living things on planet Earth, including everything from the emergence of chromosomes, to the emergence of multicellular organisms, to the emergence of human culture (see also Wilson 2012). Remarkably, in each case the transition was characterized by the same two fundamental processes: (1) a new form of cooperation with almost total interdependence among individuals (be they cells or organisms) that creates a new functional entity, and (2) a concomitant new form of communication to support this cooperation.

Why we stood up

When multicellular organisms were first expanding their internal complexity 500 million years ago, neurological systems were evolved to coordinate their behavior.

---

[25] I cannot help but wonder at what Carl Jung would have thought of Tomasello's speculations in light of these testy remarks about Freud:

> As for Freud's concept of the "superego," it is a furtive attempt to smuggle the time-honored image of Jehovah in the dress of psychological theory. For my part, I prefer to call my things by the names under which they have always been called (*Freud and Psychoanalysis*, Bollingen Series XX).

The key is *rapid and continuous* real-time communication to *all* constituents of the organism. How could such communication have been established in these first hominin group-organisms?

To appreciate the limitations of communication between animals selected at the level of individuals, it is enlightening to read the abstract from a classic article on the subject by Robert Seyfarth and Dorothy Cheney (2003) titled "Signalers and Receivers in Animal Communication":

> In animal communication natural selection favors callers who vocalize to af-fect [i.e. manipulate] the behavior of listeners and listeners who [are selected to] acquire information from vocalizations. The [emotional] mechanisms that cause a signaler to vocalize do not limit a listener's ability to extract infor-mation from the call. Whereas signalers may vocalize to change a listener's behavior, they do not call to inform others. Listeners acquire information from signalers who do not, in the human sense, intend to provide it.

In other words, in animals evolved only for the fitness of the individual, expres-sions are always manipulative, and understanding expressions is the equivalent of eavesdropping. These characteristics are opposite of the hyper-transparency in-trinsic to collective expressions.

The most fundamental fact in human evolution is that upright posture is an abso-lute requirement for a fossil to be designated a hominin. In the oldest hominin skull fossils, the extent of upright posture is determined by the forward position of the hole in the bottom of the skull (*foramen magnum*) through which the spinal cord exits. Because any orthopedic surgeon can tell you that upright posture pro-duces extreme vulnerability for injuries to the lower back, perennially among the top ER visits (Weiss, 2011), and to joints in the lower limbs, it is reasonable to conclude that the evolutionary advantages of such a costly adaptation must have been central to the functioning even of the earliest hominins.

My narrative is that from the beginning, in the first hominin species, communica-tion became the indispensable "neurological system" for the burgeoning group-organism. For the group to begin evolving teamwork coordination, the sheer vol-ume of information required to be simultaneously-and-continuously expressed-and-comprehended had to increase by many orders of magnitude. Is it not reason-able to conclude that creatures stood up to be in constant visual contact with other group members' facial and upper body gestural expressions? This would allow them to coordinate behavior in the same manner that a musical band makes small adjustments to stay in sync. This is what Darwin calls the "language of emotions" in which "expression in itself . . . is certainly of importance for the welfare of mankind." In effect, the entire body evolved into an instrument of constant mutual expression that knit together the group-organism into an organic social system.

Whether it be a high-powered negotiation or a tea party, the prototypical human configuration is a circle in which everyone can see everyone else without regard to rank. The circular megalithic culture in Britain, beginning in the Orkney Islands in northern Scotland more than six thousand years ago[26] and culminating with Stonehenge, reflects the deepest human impulses, whereas pyramidal architecture in Mesopotamia, Egypt, and Mesoamerica reflect our hierarchical ape heritage. Our individual, hierarchical, and dominance-oriented ape mind has only recently re-emerged within the span of our own species.

The early hominins

A characteristic feature of early hominins, such as the famous 3.2-million-year-old Lucy fossils, is large molar teeth (*megadontia*). Microwear studies of these teeth reveal they were evolved to grind up tough grasses and sedges (Ungar, 2017). At this stage, hominins would be a kind of herd animal, but with a big difference. Obviously, dryer colder climates in the region at that time are central here, but eating low-quality foods could also be interpreted as preserving their nascent advantage of teamwork by naturally selecting *against* disruptive competition that inevitably resulted from seeking high quality foods like meat. Of course, the hunted became very much the hunter with the arrival of our Homo genus, but, perhaps by that time, justice had become entrenched enough to immunize their organic social structure from the internal disruption of dominance seeking.

In a landmark study, an analysis of the movements of a troop of GPS-wearing baboons demonstrated that the animals actually leading the troop around had no correlation with dominance rank (Strandburg-Peshkin, 2015). Perhaps the one

---

[26] Evidence that the Neolithic Orkney Island civilization had little sense of individuality is that, after their dead were reduced to skeletons, they entombed the heads, arms, and legs each in separate chambers.

with the most friends is "pulling" them around with separation anxiety as is the case with feral dogs[27] (Bonanni, 2010). Could it be that, as dominance was suppressed in hominins, long-evolved democratic affiliative instincts emerged to predominate? The next chapter will detail the strange story of how primate dominance hierarchies reemerged to create the hybrid social system of our own species.

Another provocative fact about the early hominins has recently come to light as a result of two fossil finds in South Africa, *Australopithecus sediba* and *Homo naledi*, which both contain unusually large numbers of postcranial fossils (ribs, limbs, etc). Lee Berger, the paleoanthropologist directing these sites, noted that the same *mosaic* of skeletal features in species found elsewhere in Africa—feet, ribcage, spine, hands, shoulders—evolved at different rates, but they all were moving in the same direction. There are feet adapted to traveling long distances, pelvises for the same reason plus giving birth to larger brains, rib cages for respiratory endurance, and of course hands with opposable thumbs for constructing and manipulating tools. Berger speculates (2017) that all these species interbred, but this still begs the question of the environmental cause of the *unitary direction* of these incremental changes all evolving in different African climates. Once again, the defining mental environment shared by all hominins was that of collective intentionality.

What was it like living in one of these early hominin groups? In my imagination, I picture becoming aware of a continuous chirping sound threading up from below while hiking on a promontory high above the East African savanna three million years ago. After lying down with my binoculars to examine the vast plain beneath me, I am astonished by the sight of two groups of grass-eating apes, separated by roughly a quarter of a mile. I am charmed and fascinated to have discovered two herds, all harmlessly crouching and munching together. From the beginning, and steadily increasing, I have a profound sense that these creatures are unique. I finally see two of these three-to-four-foot tall animals (presumably mates) stand up straight and walk over to the other group to join them, but that is the least of it. It is subtle at first, but once recognized, undeniable: I become aware that the indi-

---

[27] This is so even though Range and Virányi (2014) showed that the hierarchies of dog packs are more strongly dominance based than those of wolves.

viduals in each group as well as constantly vocalizing are all simultaneously gesturing to each other. They emit a continuous emotional intensity that causes within me a growing sense of foreboding—of fear. As peaceable and closely comfortable as they are with each other, the thought occurs to me that if they discover my presence, all that harmony might instantly merge, and they could become extremely dangerous to an outsider.

So fearing for my life while fatally drawn to them, I watch them from my lofty perch. For two days, I am tortured by my inability to pin down what it is about them that both terrifies and enthralls me. Gradually I focus on how intensely in tune they are with one another, without a hint of dominance or hierarchy. Each group will be doing different things, but not at the lazy pace of chimps in a zoo or the way ordinary herd animals often react simultaneously to the environment. Then it hits me like a thunderstone.[28] The individuals in these groups are not only cooperating with one another; the entire behavior in these two groups is coordinated as if emanating from a single creature.

The Homo peoples

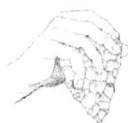

The toolmaking capacities of our ancestral species is qualitatively different from toolmaking in animals and would not have arisen in the absence of collective intentionality. The manufacture of stone tools arose and evolved into the almost universal use of the Acheulean hand ax, which remained essentially unchanged for 1.5 million years, a time of unprecedented brain growth. Although part of the progression of this early tool industry involved widely dispersed genetically mediated manual dexterity, an opposable thumb, and hand-eye coordination, there can be no doubt that the actual method of stone tool construction was spread culturally—and there is the rub.

Adaptive genetic changes in the hands and brain occur slowly, and therefore would have had time to *drift* their way into the far-flung gene pool of the various species of the Homo people. In contrast, we are used to thinking that cultural practices happen far more quickly, spread only locally and, as a result, the stone tool industry should manifest more local and temporal variation. We normally think of

---

[28] Hominin hand axes were called *thunderstones* in the middle ages. They were thought to have dropped from the sky, having been somehow produced by thunder and lightning.

these kinds of cultural practices as spreading by *imitation*, making their continuity over long distances and times fragile and subject to variation. Darwin's challenge was to construct a theory that contained potential dynamic change over time within apparently unchanging species; but the challenge of the hand ax is quite the opposite—why is there such enduring stasis in usually rapidly changing cultural transmission?

First, there is evidence that hand axes were made in groups. In *Fairweather Eden* (1998), Michael Pitts and Mark Roberts deduced by the placement of half-million-year-old stone chips uncovered in Boxgrove, England, that they had been knapped off hand axes constructed simultaneously in groups. In the context of coordinating hand ax knapping in groups and groups of groups, constant migration combined with high levels of cooperation led to homogenized construction of this tool through vast spans of time and space.

The first documented migration out of Africa was 1.8 million years ago, but there were previous migrations within Africa. Although changing climates and diets initiated migration, it most likely was unprecedented cooperation among the early Homo peoples that made them so successful. Marcus Hamilton and his associates (2009) determined through the mathematical modeling of later modern human migrations out of Africa that cooperation was the essential factor in their global success, and the same logic applies to these earlier migrations.

It is usually assumed that migration is a one-way street, forever outward bound. However, Anna Olivieri and her associates (2006) determined by means of sequencing modern human mitochondrial DNA that human migration 40 to 45 thousand years ago also consisted of significant migration back into Africa. Likely the mixing effect of back and forth migration also occurred with the early members of the genus Homo almost two million years earlier.

It seems likely these migrating groups of Homo peoples, selected almost entirely for the productivity of their relationships, had little or no sense of individuality and that kin-selected family identities were relatively weak compared to the more general and predominant bond forged by the decisive benefits of teamwork. I maintain that a central function of knapping these tools, beyond butchering animals and other speculated uses, was as a ritual bonding exercise that reflected their organic way of life in that it was led by the authority of those who knew best how it should be done.

While I can only imagine watching the early hominins from afar, I can easily place myself among these early Homo people. Crouching in a circle, we are all glancing back and forth, not merely imitating one another's work, but watching for strokes made with the authority of how it should be and always had been done. We all instinctively know the familiar rectitude of wisdom flashing alternatively among us, making small adjustments with constant mutual recognition until general specifications are satisfied: the precise technique of striking, the proper size and form, sharpened all around the edges.

The essential unity of these far-flung artifacts bears witness to the collective sources of their creation rendered deeply from within the same sacred way of life. There was no planning or knowing outside the moment of being submerged within the midst of their communal movements, one leading right on to the next in a rhythm of stones striking stones that were the sounds and motions all from within thousands of tiny, separate groups all animated by a single, eternal Will. It is meaningless to assert that these people were religious, but it could be said they lived their lives inside the mind of a naturally evolved deity.

Whether it be from one day, week, or century on into the next, the memory of what to do and when to do it was not stored in any individual brain. Rather, this knowledge was mixed into and among a given group—and all groups—in bits and pieces, which, when the moment arose, fell together in collective animation. Diffusing through time and space and linked by long repeating chains of unbroken mutual experience, this hallowed ritual, the emblem of a sacred tribe, scattered far and wide out into their diaspora from Africa out and across the vastness of Eurasia. Although individuals drifted from one group to another, small bands dissolved, and new ones reconstituted, these diurnal chains of communal functioning wove an unbroken fabric for 50 thousand generations across the expanse of entire continents.

Big brains

An often-cited study of primate species by British anthropologist and evolutionary psychologist Robin Dunbar (1992) demonstrates the bigger the size of the species' average group membership, the larger the brain. "Machiavellian intelligence" is a term used to describe the competitive ability to read an opponent's mind, which, in a hierarchy, is informed by knowing everyone's rank at a given time. The bigger the group, the bigger the brain needed to keep track of a large, fluid hierarchy. Projecting from his work with primates, Dunbar calculated that later Homo peoples' groups would have grown to 150 members while evolving the big brains we now have.

However, when Dunbar began to study what correlated to large brain size in non-primate mammals, much to his initial dismay, he found the correlation was to monogamy rather than group size (2007). He describes the cognitively demanding behavior in monogamous pair-bonds as "active synchronization," recognized that bonding is an "emotional experience," and that "language is a notoriously poor medium for describing our inner emotional experiences." Acknowledging the power of empathy as a tool in understanding emotion, he adds, "Intuitively, we know what we mean by bondedness because we experience it ourselves, and we recognize it when it happens."

Brain growth in the Homo peoples reflected increasing effectiveness in collectively distilling on the fly the essential narratives in sequences of environmental events matched with those collective responses that led to success, for example in stalking prey. Language expanded in the lateral brain lobes. Stanford neuro-endocrinologist Robert M. Sapolsky in *Behave: The Biology of Humans at Our Best and Worst* (2017) defines frontal lobe function as, "Doing the harder thing when it's the right thing to do." Sapolsky lays out evidence that the fundamental "default" of human social behavior is trust, and that the amygdala, the brain structure concerned with anxiety, fear and rage, is sensitive to unfairness and is involved in applying justice when needed:

> The amygdala . . . plays a logical role in social and emotional decision making. In the Ultimatum Game, an economic game involving two players, the first makes an offer as to how to divide a pot of money, which the other player either accepts or rejects. If the latter, neither gets anything. Research shows that rejecting an offer is an emotional decision, triggered by anger at a lousy offer and the desire to punish. The more the amygdala activation in the second player after an offer, the more likely the rejection. People with damaged amygdalae are atypically generous in the Ultimatum Game and don't increase rejection rates if they start receiving unfair offers. . . . these findings suggest that the amygdala injects implicit distrust and vigilance into social decision making. All thanks to learning. . . . The investigators involved state: "The generosity in the trust game of our BLA [amygdala]-damaged subjects might be considered pathological altruism, in the sense that *inborn altruistic*

behaviors [italics mine] have not, due to BLA damage, been un-learned through negative social experience."

Sapolsky goes on to explain that among the inputs to the amygdala is a region in the prefrontal cortex called the *insula,* which is activated when one tastes or smells something disgusting. This area is also activated by morally objectionable behavior: "Someone does something lousy and selfish to you in a game, and the extent of insular and amygdaloid activation predicts how much outrage you feel and how much revenge you take. This is all about sociality—the insula and amygdala don't activate if it's a computer that has stabbed you in the back." So the amygdala is intricately responsive to moral sensibilities.

The excavation of Urmensch

I have long thought depictions of the face of our ancestral hominin species have been too apelike. There is very little science on what hominin faces looked like, only the skulls beneath the faces. With this in mind I commissioned German illustrator Jürgen Willbarth to draw an image of what he began calling an *urmensch* (ancient man), a name which I adopted.

He first drew the composite sketch shown here from a half dozen pictures of hominin heads fashioned by paleo-sculptors informed by fossil skulls. I call this sketch an "easel" in the letter below, written to him in German, and then I proceed to specify what I had in mind:

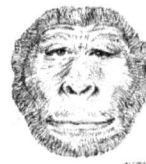

> Sehr geehrter Herr Willbarth,
>
> Excellent! We now have an easel upon which to work. I would like to see in this face the etched effects of a life of care and concern around the eyes; remember, this is a face no one has ever seen or even conceived of before. The expression around the mouth is too lighthearted. I want a careworn expression (but not at all depressed or sad) to reflect a life of responsibility. Give the face the lines of <u>character</u>. These were very serious, kind, and compassionate people, far more so than we. Vanity and pride did not yet exist.
>
> Please allow me to briefly summarize for you what I have determined about the evolution of the human face. For our ancestral species it was exclusively an instrument of communication. Most animals do not have a face in the human sense, because it is not in their interest to

communicate much of anything but aggression. Apes have the beginnings of a face principally to communicate dominance or submission. The human face became flattened in the front, like an information billboard (which is what we have in your first rendering). Right from the beginning, our ancestral species evolved a communication system (language) in which there was sustained signaling and receiving in order to achieve a running consensus about two burning issues: justice and truth.

The function of the modern human face has diverged, in part, from that of our ancestors. Our faces are also used as an organ of display, like a peacock's tail. We have evolved a superimposed "layer" reflecting our passion for vanity. That is why modern faces look so childlike—particularly female faces with retained baby fat, and reduced noses and jaws in order to resemble cute children. So the objective here is to excavate out from under our present baby-face the finely chiseled and thoroughly functional dignity that was the countenance of our noble ancestors.

With regard for your skills,

John Wylie

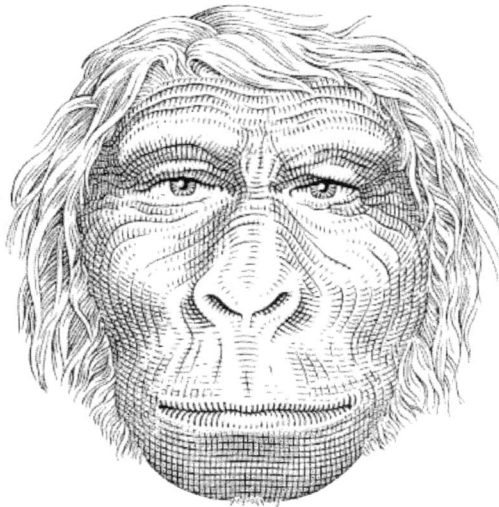

Urmensch

PART THREE

DESTINY'S CHILDREN

CHAPTER 9

MODERN HUMANS:
THE ENIGMA OF VANITY

The audience

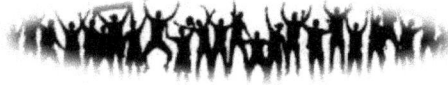

Forty-five years ago, while in my psychiatric residency, I moonlighted at D.C. General Hospital's emergency room. I never knew who would come in the doors down there at the General. The "White House cases" were a staple, a motley collection of characters pulled off the fence surrounding the presidential residence. One evening is etched in my mind. I received the usual call at about midnight from the nurse, who told me they had a "doozy." The on-call room was quite a distance from the ER, and when I turned a corner, I could see a bit of a hubbub at the end of the long corridor.

After everything finally settled down, the patient was more than eager to spill out the inner details of the day's adventures. The character I am about to inhabit omnisciently is, like the protagonist of T. S. Eliot's poem "The Love Song of J. Alfred Prufrock," an average person anxiously adjusted to a narrow modern life.

Early that morning, this usually nondescript gentleman woke up and, I am here to tell you, he felt G*R*E*A*T! Most of all he felt an enormous amount of energy, which William Blake described as "eternal delight." He leapt out of bed, his mind racing. His belly was full of laughter and fun. He imagined he had a large, appreciative audience anticipating with collective bated breath what in the world he might do next. "Wait till they see my next move! They'll be rolling in the aisles! They'll love it—but first I need some cash." He hurried to the bank and struck up conversations with several bemused passersby while waiting for the bank to open. "I need a new car and I want to pay cash for it today," he told the banker, who was captivated by the utter confidence of his ebullient mood.

Next, he drew a crowd at the Cadillac showroom as he theatrically insisted that he buy the model off the showroom floor. He was in a hurry, wanting to pursue whatever wonderful activity he would do next (which shifted with every passing moment). As he got behind the wheel, he suddenly thought, "It's a beautiful day. A great day to go out to the beach, and who knows what great, fun things might happen!" As he pulled out into traffic, though, he saw a costume shop; unable to resist the riotous possibilities it might hold for him and his hoard of watchers, he took a U-turn, screeched the car to a halt, and rushed inside.

When I first reached the ER, this fulminant figure was surrounded by three or four of DC's finest. He was being picked up for "disorderly conduct." Before me was a fifty-plus-year-old balding man in a rumpled blue Superman costume, the cape twisted around to the front like a large red bib. The pièce de résistance was that he wore a necklace comprised of small plastic breasts.

This person was in the grip of an acute manic episode.

Mania as a fossil

The idea that mania is a pathological exaggeration of sexual display epitomized by the peacock's tail occurred to me while reading psychologist Geoffrey Miller's *The Mating Mind: How Sexual Choice Shaped the Evolution of Human Nature* (2000). Once the evolutionary psychoanalytic significance of mania is contemplated, its connection with sexual selection becomes evident. Although there are ubiquitous examples of sexual display in nature, there are no animal models for sustained states of pathologically hyperactive sexual display as in manic disorder, an illness that contains the feedback reverberated essence of all that is unique to our own peculiar species.

The specific entity of mania in bipolar disorder, previously known as manic depression, is often obscured by its almost invariable association with depression. I have explained that in the other two major depression illnesses, the brain-shutdown symptoms of lethargy and lack of initiative could either be reactive, or a direct freezing response to the primary hyperactive-anxiety component of these illnesses. Whereas in the depression illnesses these "negative" symptoms are mixed in with the active component, in bipolar disorder the actively pathological manic component is manifested by itself, serially and separated in time from the presumably reactive shutdown symptoms of depression that normally follow the manic phase. Therefore, it is the hyperactive, manic component of bipolar disorder that reveals the fossilized clues as to what is exclusively modern in our long hominin evolution.

Before plunging into the treasure trove of insights about why mania reveals so much about modern human nature, it is important to state clearly that bipolar disorder is a devastating illness. Although the manic phase is usually experienced as euphoric, its consequences can be disastrous, not only for the patient but for the family. The associated depressive phase, which almost always lasts much longer than the manic phase, is exceedingly painful to the patient. As the illness progresses, there is often a cruel mixing of the manic and depressive components producing an excruciatingly agitated state of chronically *racing thoughts* mixed with anxiety. Like schizophrenia, when not in an acute episode, it is appropriate to refer to these individuals as living with their illness and not just passive sufferers. However, untreated, a patient with bipolar disorder may withdraw into a chronic siege mentality of paranoid grandiosity.

Mercifully, bipolar disorder has an array of effective treatments. The first "miracle" drug in psychiatry was Lithium, a simple salt substitute. Like nearly all other psychiatric medications, an astute serendipitous observation led to its use in humans. Dr. John Cade (1912-1980) in Melbourne, Australia, noted in 1949 that an injection of lithium had a calming effect on guinea pigs.

Mania is a disabling disease that reveals much about our emotional makeup. The innovation resulting in the evolution of our own species was the development of an intensely positive sensation elicited when others admire us. The endless nature of *Homo sapiens'* hunger for attention from one another distinguishes our species. The powerful drive to seek the attention of an *audience* has resulted in the development of an endless variety of species-specific behaviors tantamount to competitive sexual display. The pervasiveness of this strong proclivity in humans renders us all at once brilliantly creative, cruel, and absurd. Ancient biblical texts distilled these qualities into a single word: *vanity*.

The language connection

There have been occasions when I have been temporarily drawn from my role as a physician into stunned fascination by the linguistic performance of a patient in the throes of a manic illness. All manner of rhetorical flourishes and beautifully constructed phrases may pour out in a torrent. Often there is a magnetic quality to this verbal virtuosity, the meaning of which can constitute a brilliantly creative *flight of ideas*. In the biography by Sylvia Nasar of the mathematician John Nash, *A Beautiful Mind: The Life of Mathematical Genius and Nobel Laureate John Nash* (1998), a visitor relates the following incident at the McLean Hospital in Boston, where Nash was hospitalized for schizophrenia:

> Robert Lowell, the poet, walked in, manic as hell. He sees this very pregnant woman. He looks at her and starts quoting the begat sequences in the Bible. Then he started spinning quotes with the word "anointed." He decided to lecture us on the meaning of "anointed" in all the ways it was used in the King James Version of the Bible. In the end I decided that every word in the English language was a personal friend of his (Simon & Schuster edition, p. 260).

Here Lowell's poetic flight is an emotional fossil of the singular passion that our own species brings to the hominin tribe.

Vital to dating a fossil is careful evaluation of the surrounding geologic strata in which the fossil is found. The extraordinary hyperactivity of the intricately complex structure (syntax) of spoken language is one of the most central and dramatic behavioral manifestations in mania and is the equivalent of such a stratum.

Linguists are chronically irritated by amateurs like me impinging on their highly specialized field, particularly when it comes to evolution. For that reason, my forays into language are closely chaperoned by recognized authorities. The first generalization is that the syntactical aspect of language is complex and cognitively demanding. Therefore, as Ray Jackendoff, a prominent linguist at Tufts University, puts it in his *Foundations of Language: Brain, Meaning, Grammar, Evolution* (2002, p. 427), syntax "has the feel of a relatively late innovation," that is, a recent evolutionary development.

As described in the previous chapter, hominins almost certainly had robustly expressive language that involved sharing their collective intentions, which set them apart from all other primates. But it is the byzantine complexity of grammar that has propelled us into another sphere. It is my conviction that the verbal, syntactic gymnastics that regularly accompany mania fix the disorder as deriving from a suite of normal behaviors that were the principal adaptations in the evolution of our *Homo sapiens* species.

There is also a link between spoken language and the idea that the evolution of *Homo sapiens* involved sexual selection. In *The Descent of Man, and Selection in Relation to Sex* (1871), Darwin associated the concept of sexual selection with vocal language in human evolution. Drawing on the example in nature of male birdsong, Darwin wrote:

> The impassioned orator, bard, or musician, when with his various tones and cadences, he excites the strongest emotions in his hearers, little suspects that he uses the same means by which, at an extremely remote period, his half-human ancestors aroused each other's passions, during their mutual court-ship and rivalry.

In his erudite but highly readable book *The Evolution of Language* (2010), linguist W. Tecumseh Fitch supports the association between the origin of human language and song:

> The core virtue of the musical protolanguage hypothesis is its logical expla-nation of the design features shared by song and spoken language, namely the use of the vocal/auditory channel to generate complex, hierarchically structured signals that are learned and shared across generations.

Darwin's original idea of associating vocal language with sexual selection remains alive and well today. For example, think back to when you were going through puberty, at the peak of your sexuality, and remember how utterly enraptured you were with popular music.

A species of hypersexual hominin kids

For those who doubt that emotions can undergo evolution, the fifty-year experi-ment run by Lyudmila Trut in Russia, recently detailed in *How to Tame a Fox (and Build a Dog)* (Dugatkin and Trut, 2017), is edifying. She attracted worldwide attention for her pioneering study of the domestication of silver foxes. Selection for calm temperament in foxes brought along with it a suite of traits associated with dogs, including strong attachments to humans, social intelligence, playful behavior, tail wagging, physiological changes in hormones affecting reproduction, and even physical changes associated with dogs, such as floppy ears, curly tails, and colored patches. Several of these traits indicate that the genes initiating ma-turity have been turned off by domestication.

Many scholars have put forward the possibility that a process of self-domestication initiated the transition into our own species (Gibbons, 2014). It is certainly plausible that dog-like (self-) domestication merely kick-started our own evolution by instilling preference for the youthful behavior and looks that are linked to calmer temperaments, as in dogs and foxes. Just as dogs are playful wolf-pups for life, modern humans are playful hominin-kids for life. No matter how it began, sexual selection transformed those initial changes into elaborate self-display behaviors, such as the beautiful 35,000-year-old paintings in the Chauvet Pont d'Arc Cave in Ardèche, France, that thoroughly mark us as a species.

Yale ornithologist Richard Prum published a significant book in 2017 titled *The Evolution of Beauty: How Darwin's Forgotten Theory of Mate Choice Shapes the Animal World - and Us*. Dr. Prum is a first-class field naturalist in the tradition of Charles Darwin, Edward Wilson (ants), and Thomas Seeley (bees, 2010). In *The Evolution of Beauty,* he dusts off Darwin's theory of sexual selection, clearly explains it, and pointedly dispatches all the *adaptationist* proposals that sexually selected traits must, in some circuitous way, confer fitness and survival benefits. Prum embraces Darwin's often ignored conclusion that the mere desire for beauty—pleasure itself—is the driving force behind the aesthetically pleasing aspects not only of our bodies, but also our temperaments.

Prum makes a compelling case that female mate choice plays a decisive role in diminishing the dominance mentality in human males, and he assigns desire for autonomy as the motivation. I have proposed that this same dynamic played a fundamental role in founding our hominin tribe. I am indebted to Dr. Prum for the authority that his erudition brings to bear on redeeming Darwin's most profound insight specifically relating to human evolution.

There is paleontological evidence for sexual selection. What makes early human fossils recognizably modern is that they come from individuals who would have been physically attractive to us: slender with childlike skulls, the result of a process known as *neoteny*. This view was recently buttressed by fossils found in West African Morocco (instead of the usual sites in the East African rift valley or South Africa), which were dated at roughly 300,000 years (Hublin, 2017). These fossils are now thought to be derived from early members of our own species due to—among other traits—their "delicate cheek-bones." However, these skulls have an elongated braincase, like prior hominin species, which evolved into the globular shaped head with a small-and-divided brow ridge above a small face that is characteristic of modern humans. It is a spare and reasonable explanation to assume that these transformations were the result of sexual selection in the direction of the appearance of a juvenile skull. All this begs the question of whether the stupendous intelligence that we have brought to the hominin table has largely been motivated by vanity.

Evidence for sexual selection abounds in modern humans. Retention of juvenile features that result in more youthful-looking adults makes those adults more appealing to the opposite sex. Women are markedly neotenic (retaining youthful traits into adulthood), with reduced noses and jaws (although jutting jaws in general are a modern addition). Yet onto their infantilized anatomies, most evident in puberty, human females have added exaggerated sexual characteristics, such as rounded breasts, which, in contrast to all other primates, are present even when the females are not lactating. And let us not ignore the growth of penises in puberty (mainly thicker than those of chimps including the bulbous end, called the *glans*) that human females have selected along the way.

It is common for patients with mania to be hypersexual, and indeed, this trait exists in the normal array of modern human motivations. Sometimes when I look at a picture of Freud in one of his thoroughly grim poses, I search for a little twinkle in his eye, wondering whether he got a kick out of scandalizing the Victorian world with the fact that their minds were chock full of sexual motivation. This promiscuous tendency in humans is underlain and modulated, however, by our six-million-year legacy of monogamy. The dynamic between promiscuous sexuality and monogamy, played out in countless soap operas, is a backdoor introduction to the theme of the next chapter, in which we will explore the normal interaction between the old hominin mind and the new modern-human mind, revealed by mania.

However, it is not our hypersexuality nor our sexually selected physical traits that set modern humans apart from all other creatures; it is the powerful motivation that generates our prodigiously protean behavioral displays, which is *the desire to be desired*, whether male or female. This impulse to be admired encompasses a global motivation in *Homo sapiens* behavior and is in stark contrast to the motivations that had previously been evolving for millions of years.

Freud had a concept of global sexuality that he called narcissism, which relates not only to inordinate love of oneself, but also to the desire to be admired by others. Narcissism has been a concept that psychoanalysts have struggled with since Freud's time. It has had pathological implications for the curiously straitlaced psychoanalytic ideal of psychosexual maturity. However, in the 1970s, Viennese-born American psychoanalyst Hans Kohut attempted to rehabilitate the reputation of narcissism by proposing that the personality possesses a *self-system* (separate from the anxiety-driven ego-system) within which the nurturing of narcissism in the child is vital to achieve a healthy self-esteem in the well-adjusted adult (self-psychology). In fact, when we in the "audience" are evaluating the behavior of others, we accept that all motivations for the good of the group are tinged with narcissism because we have co-evolved a discerning taste and predilection for these displays—for charisma, charm, and the mysterious quality of talent.

Nevertheless, the term *narcissism* continues to have a negative connotation. So hereafter I will refer to this entirely normal human emotion-and-motivation simply as *self-display* to emphasize that its goal is getting others to love us and that loving ourselves (for good reasons) is normally a great way to accomplish that goal; that is, it is part of the display. I call it self-display and not sexual display to emphasize that this uniquely human desire to be desired is directed not only to the opposite sex, but also to a nonspecific social audience. This imaginary audience tends to expand well beyond one's own group. In the words of Shakespeare, "All the world's a stage."

In *Homo sapiens* the sexually selected desire for self-display took the lead role in shaping the desire for these displays in the audience, instead of vice versa (as in birds). It is as if peacocks started to influence the selection of their tails by developing sexy sales pitches about the tail's special virtues. As in all sexual selection, genetic underpinnings of the desire for beauty becomes linked to the genetic underpinnings of the desire to be desired for being or doing something beautiful. However, unlike peahens and peacocks, modern humans are simultaneously both the desirer and the desired.

Indeed, our minds are comprised of capacities determined by motivations involving both actor and object of the action, and this has much to do with expansive human consciousness and linguistic virtuosity. We are at once the seer and the seen, condemner and condemned, lover and loved. However, because human evolution left us so fraught with these condensed motivations, our minds are also vulnerable to the unraveling of emotion into the spinning feedback scream of mental illness.

Symbols and culture

Body decoration, like wearing a necklace of pierced shells, is seen by scholars as an advance in the cognitive ability to create *symbols* enabled by fortuitous genetic mutations (the "cognitive revolution"). The shell necklace is a symbol if it stands for something else, like belonging to a group or conveying social status. I propose that wearing jewelry only secondarily became symbolic, and that a more plausible explanation for its emergence is as a natural response to the simultaneous desire for—and the desire to be desired for—beauty. The principle in play here is that, when there is a will, the will finds a way.

One dimension of the sexually selected response to beauty, in this case a beautiful shell, is to find it attractive and perhaps pick it up. But then, the other linked motivational component is that it is you (and not the shell) that wishes to be desired for being beautiful. The first step in the resolution of this dilemma is to *possess* the shell. However, although everyone needs to know that the shell belongs to you, what is the sense of owning it if you do not show it off? So, ardently drawn by these vain desires, how much brain power would it take to figure out how to display that pretty shell by poking a hole in it and fastening it around your neck with a reed? And once a couple of people started doing it, many more would have started imitating it, like an early fashion craze.

Tellingly, one of Kohut's principal observations is that the communication of esteem during therapy involves *mirroring*, in which a patient imitates a healthy positive self-regard in the therapist. An important feature of self-display behavior is that it may effectively be transmitted through imitation or mirroring. The ease of mirroring contrasts with the much more emotional, drawn-out process of identification employed by our hominin ancestors. The process of identification is disabled and exposed in schizophrenia and is reflected in the stability of hand ax construction described in the last chapter. Learning by imitation is a central element that led to the emergence of rapidly evolving culture, which is the thesis of *Darwin's Unfinished Symphony: How Culture Made the Human Mind* (2017) by

Kevin Laland, a senior authority on the relationship between culture and evolution.

Key to understanding the benefits of vanity is to focus on the emotion that animates self-display behavior. This emotion can be summed up in the word *desire*. We *Homo sapiens* are the primates who desire. And what is it that is desired? Each other. *Homo sapiens* constantly, relentlessly, and irrepressibly desire each other. This desire resulted in the overall strengthening of bonds between individuals and induced a motivational force that drew together larger and larger intercommunicating groups for which there is genetic evidence.[29]

The formation of culture, which is the natural selection of know-how across generations, is a major milestone in the history of human life. The emergence of human desire coalesced critical population densities that led to the emergence of culture, off and on for a long time before taking off about 40,000 years ago. My position is that human culture resurrected our ape mind along with the structure of dominance hierarchies in the process of amalgamating groups of groups. Artifacts, long used as ornaments, adopted symbolic functions, like group identity or status (with no cognitive leaps necessary). Beneath our species' sordid history of chronic war, it is boundlessly creative desire born of sexual selection that is the core animating instinct we modern humans have affixed, as if an ornament, upon the profound legacy of justice bequeathed by our ancestral species.

The earliest cultural artifacts associated with modern humans date from around 100,000 years ago and are found in both north and south Africa as well as along early migration routes east of the Mediterranean. These artifacts consist primarily of shells and pierced beads clearly used as body ornaments and red ocher, a natural clay earth pigment whose exact use is unknown. A good guess is that it decorated the body, a use that continues in regions of modern Africa.

---

[29]Comparative genome sequencing on Neanderthals from about 60,000 years ago (Prüfer, 2017) demonstrated that they were "highly inbred, . . . lived in small groups, and had lower genetic diversity." This is compared to the genomes of four 34,000-year-old *Homo sapiens* from Eastern Russia (Sikora, 2017). Although from the same kinship group, their genomes . . . "were not very closely related. Thus, these people may represent a single social group that was part of a larger mating network, similar to contemporary hunter-gatherers. The lack of close inbreeding might help to explain the survival advantage of anatomically modern humans."

It was natural for gold to become the most valuable commodity for humans because it is far more durable and its luster does not tarnish, making it an ideal body adornment. Think of the enduring gleam of Tutankhamen's three nested coffins (Egyptian gods were believed to have gold skin) and the stacks of ingots in the coffers at Fort Knox. Underscoring the use that underlies the value humans place on gold is the fact that 52 percent of it continues to be used for jewelry (2017, World Gold Council). For evidence of the power of self-display in today's electronic world, one need only consider the influence and market value of social media.

Romance and rage

Grandiosity is the manic symptom that expresses more than just an inflated sense of self-importance and authority. The word describes the impulse not just to do one's duty and pull the oar, but to have everyone sit up and take notice: "Now, that's someone special, not the ordinary sort of rower but a true original." Encouragingly, there is often a broad magnanimous streak couched within the symptoms of mania. For example, within the sanctuary of my humble clinical office, vast entrepreneurial schemes have been disclosed, including at least one vision of curing cancer. A reigning emperor of the world (benevolent) came to see me, as well as an aspiring messiah. The feeling of mania is the excitement of serious celebrity, of being watched and admired by the multitudes with more than a touch of awe. Around the time of the American Bicentennial, a man had the gallant aspiration of single-handedly constructing a ship named *Independence* and triumphantly sailing it up the Potomac. The impulses revealed by mania are the source of human enterprise, vision, imagination, and creativity.

Often, after a manic episode, leaving aside the agony of the depression that usually follows, the patient looks back with a sense of wistfulness, like recollecting an ill-fated love affair. In milder cases of *hypomania*, the spouse often needs to corroborate that a period of time that the patient considered positive was actually one during which there was loss of judgment: an extravagant villa was purchased overseas; night after night, ancient insects trapped in amber were feverishly bought on eBay; or he or she merely talked too much to anyone who would listen and was uncharacteristically expansive, with an incremental loss of social propriety.

One can easily understand the link between mania and genius in people who seem to be chronically in highly productive states of so-called subclinical *hypomania* but who remain well within the bounds of mental health. To pick one of the most visible examples, Winston Churchill, given to prolonged bouts of depression, was probably in a hypomanic state all during World War II; for example, he is said to have sashayed around the White House without any clothes on while visiting, hardly slept at all, and consumed large quantities of alcohol, which is associated with all forms of mania.

A view of mania through the lens of Darwin's theory of sexual selection affords insight into human avarice, as wild spending sprees are one of mania's consistent symptoms. Buying a fancy sports car may serve the same purpose as those ancient shell necklaces, and, indeed, at the heart of the profit motive lies a vision not of power but romance, like that evoked by the gold rush and wildcatting for oil in the Wild West.

For us daffy moderns, romance + power = status. Buying fun things is a shortcut to feeling self-esteem. The degree to which these buys are regarded as, let us say, cool, is the degree to which the purchase has achieved its sexually selected evolutionary function—which is simply to have fun. Mania, like all mental illnesses, is irreducibly social.

Unfortunately, the other side of the highly goal-driven state of mania is that intense states of *narcissistic rage* can be the response when these inflated goals are frustrated, and the rage can metastasize into dangerous paranoia. A patient who in health was a delightful person with a balanced family life when he stopped taking lithium passed through the euphoric phase into an embattled paranoid state, and barricaded himself in his home. Mania reveals an ominous dark side to the strictly modern human component of our nature.

The ego

The motivation for self-display, which is part of virtually all aspects of modern human striving, places a different light on the Freudian ego. Sigmund Freud cast the ego as a mediator between the superego's inhibitions demanded by society and the (primate) id's antisocial impulses.

To me, Freud's concept of ego resembles what philosopher Gilbert Ryle (1949) termed "the ghost in the machine," referring to the natural and widespread assumption that there is a little person or *homunculus* in our minds pulling the strings. Freud envisioned the ego as a rational (and purely defensive) diplomat, on the one hand (Charlie Chaplin) negotiating with the superego, and on the other (Woody Allen) bargaining with the id; but at the same time the ego is almost completely dependent on either the superego or id for any motivational energy at all. Nevertheless, since the Enlightenment, Western Culture has adopted the Freudian ego as an archetypal mythic hero: "I act rationally, therefore I am."

The ego that emerged in *Homo sapiens* has its own sexualized agenda, not just limited forms of sexual display as in birds, but a vastly expanded motivation to display in many different ways the special status of the individual self. This definition is more akin to a toned-down-and-widened version of what is meant by saying someone has a "big ego." Step back and consider how human it is for everyone to dress up the bare-bones reality of oneself by adding a few harmless "stretchers" to the truth—a little psychological makeup and a spiritual shoe shine—enhancing one's appearance to others. In *The River of Consciousness* (2017—published after his death), Oliver Sacks describes our self-identities as memory residues we constantly reweave into a dramatic narrative about ourselves. Occasionally asked by a patient what I thought of the vanity exposed by the frankness of our conversation, my answer was always the same: "It's only human."

The principal consequence of this re-conception of ego is the recognition that the human drive to seek this purely individual pleasure, vanity, as revealed by mania, was evolved after six million years of evolution. During all that time, obedience to the authority of groups was motivated by aversion to social fears. Clearly, vain behaviors are driven by individuals pursuing a different and often conflicting agenda from long-evolved collective behaviors for the good-of-groups.

We *Homo sapiens* emerged from our hominin base with a new agency of the mind, an *ego-mind* focused on childlike playful happiness. This individual ego was then naturally selected to interact and integrate itself with the old communal mind for the spectacular benefits of functioning together, but at the cost of mental illness. Whereas intrinsic to the old mind is the suppression of the ape mind, the new mind of the *I* evolved to function actively with the old mind of the *we*. "I think, therefore I am" becomes in light of this calculus, "We think, therefore I know I am."

CHAPTER 10

TWO HUMAN MINDS

Light will be thrown

When I first read Darwin's treatises as a young psychiatrist working in a prison, I typed out the following quotation and placed it in my wallet, where it remains:

> In the distant future I see open fields for far more important researches. Psychology will be based on a new foundation, that of the necessary acquirement of each mental power and capacity by gradation. Light will be thrown on the origin of man and his history (*On the Origin of Species*).

The stage has been set to demonstrate the power of this two-mind paradigm to render more intelligible our own most astounding and unique capacities: self-awareness leading to reflective thought, and the vast complexity of spoken language. Then this same light cast out from mental illness is cast back into the darkness that continues to isolate and stigmatize those who live with it. Thus illuminated, we recognize that they are *just like us only more so.*

Language

In Chapter 8, I discussed how the human capacity to share information and intentions contrasts with animals that are stingy and manipulative in their communications. We humans are shameless blabbermouths, constantly competing to bend each other's ears. A stark indication of collective intentionality's importance for humans is that the darkest portion of our eyes, the iris, is much smaller than it is in apes. This allows us to be constantly transparent about the direction in which we are looking. That's why quarterbacks sometimes wear tinted visors. Apes' irises are so large it is not possible to discern where they are looking because in a competitive fitness scenario, individuals evolve to conceal their intentions.

Tomasello (1999) underscores a telling capacity of children to learn that verbs like "kick" (described as "verb islands") do not have to be tied to a specific individual doing the kicking, but can be understood as a disconnected, general activity. Pre-*Homo sapiens* language was not attached to individuals, but holistically referred to group activities in which they all took part interchangeably.

Although a great deal is known about grammar and syntax, linguist W. Tecumseh Fitch calls semantics—the mystery of how meaning is understood in language—the "Wild West" of linguistic theory (2010). This problem melts away when one thinks about the old mind. The deadly serious meaning of the old mind for six million years had been restricted to a single purpose: the good of the group. Fitch credits the philosopher Paul Grice (1975) with simplifying the issue of meaning in language through a general set of rules, or "maxims," for conversation when language is on duty—and not, as Ludwig Wittgenstein (1953, ¶38) characterized it, "on vacation" playing games, which is the province of our new mind.

Grice's maxims are an exhaustive set of rules of conduct for what and how to communicate for a species shaped by the selection of individuals for the good-of-the-group, that is, group selection. The meaning of serious human conversation is about the good of a group. If you are in a leadership position of any kind, I recommend that you copy down these rules and hand them out to your employees with a note that, if they follow them all, they will definitely get a promotion.

Grice's Maxims (1975)

<u>Overall</u>: Be cooperative. Be informative.

I. <u>Maxims of Quantity</u>:
  1. Make your contributions as informative as is required.
  2. Do not make your contributions more informative than required.

II. <u>Maxims of Quality</u>:
<u>Supermaxim</u>: Try to make your contribution one that is true.
  1. Do not say what you believe is false.
  2. Do not say that for which you lack evidence.

III. <u>Maxims of Relation</u>: Be relevant.

IV. <u>Maxims of manner</u>: <u>Supermaxim</u>: Be perspicuous [transparent].
  1. Avoid obscurity of expression.
  2. Avoid ambiguity.
  3. Be brief.
  4. Be orderly

So sharing group intentions, and the understanding of actions as detached from individuals and for the good of the group, are properties of the old mind. The key function of the old mind is to disseminate interpersonal rules. The old mind is rooted in what we refer to as *character*. Character is anchored in collective social norms. First and foremost, there are the foundational 'Thou Shalt Nots' of justice and morality, essential for close coordination of within and between monogamous groups. Then, branching out in our own genus Homo are intricate conditional rules of ever more complex hunting and gathering as an organically coordinated group, everyone passionately gesturing and vocalizing while intently listening to one another, all day, every day through the millennia. The old mind is a machine that generates communal rules continuously communicated and conserved across generations, the legacy of millions of years of natural selection for the collective will not only to survive, but to thrive.

Having described the properties of human language inherited by the old mind, I now turn to the new mind. As already noted, in *The Descent of Man and Selection in Relation to Sex*, Darwin invented the concept of sexual selection and then related it to the evolution of vocal language (such as singing) in humans, an idea supported by linguist Fitch.

So here are the beginnings of an outline of the underlying emotional dynamics of human language: the interaction between: (1) the stern, maturely evolved and collectively maintained rule-making scaffolding of grammar, and (2) the ever more intricate structures of creatively artful songs sung by young people to one another, some of which catch on and spread far and wide. Darwin's genius glows in his summary definition of language as the "instinctive tendency to acquire an art."

In a 2002 paper in the journal *Science*, three eminent linguists (Marc Hauser, Noam Chomsky, and W. Tecumseh Fitch) agreed (at least briefly) that the unique property of modern language is the ability to embed multiple phrasal and clausal statements within the larger context of sentences: "This essay, which was written by a psychiatrist who loves to speculate about the big questions in life, could go on forever in an infinite number of directions." The statements, "This essay was written by a psychiatrist," "The psychiatrist loves to speculate," and others are embedded in the sentence "This essay could go on forever."

Chimpanzees that have been linguistically drilled by scientists all their lives cannot start a sentence in one direction, switch gears to embed the equivalent of another sentence (let alone two or more) within it, and then have the cognitive wherewithal or (more to the point) the *inclination* to complete the suspended initial sentence. By contrast, with our two minds, humans can simultaneously (1) hold on to the intention of the whole sentence with the scaffolding our old, rule-making mind, while (2) our new mind is motivated to embellish this linguistic structure with modifying clauses, adjectives and adverbs, some of which catch on to ebb and flow over time.

From the outset, hominin language has been distinguished by the reality that the source of its (old mind) intentions lay outside the individuals who speak "through" the authority of language that exists in the relational realm of spirit. As exquisitely put by Martin Buber in *I and Thou* (1958):

> Spirit is word. And even as verbal speech may first become word in the brain of man and then become sound in his throat, although both are merely refractions of the true event because in truth language does not reside in man but man stands in language and speaks out of it—so it is with all words, all spirit.

Being conscious of being conscious

Most thinking about self-awareness is constrained by two assumptions: 1) the mind is confined within the individual, and 2) emotions are secondary to cognitions. For example, renowned emotion researcher and author Joseph LeDoux in *The Deep History of Ourselves* (2019) states that, ". . . in my model, all emotions are cognitively assembled states of autonoetic[30] consciousness" (page 336). Freed from these constraints, a simpler explanation emerges.

In human evolution, two successively evolved configurations of social structure, comprised only of collective emotions and motivations, are the looms upon which the cognitions of our two minds have been woven. In his book bearing the same title (1999), Antonio Damasio's definition of consciousness is simply "the feeling

---

[30] *Autonoetic* is another word for self-aware. Note that the "auto-" prefix linguistically precludes my claim that the individual self (what I call ego) is immersed in a collective mentality.

of what happens." What is added to the inner feelings of our individual intentions when they engage our collective intentions is the feeling of *awareness* and *knowing*.

The task of being human is the balanced regulation between private intentions inside us and collective intentions in which we are mentally immersed. Awareness of our willfulness occurs when these private aspirations encounter the willfulness of the more ancient social sphere, long evolved as our felt collective human core—our soul. At the instant of this encounter, private aspirations "go public" and become *known* to us in the collective mental context. We modern humans continuously publicize our private feelings to ourselves so they can be "on deck" and ready to display.

Neuroscientist Benjamin Libet performed a classic experiment on free will titled "Unconscious Cerebral Initiative and the Role of Conscious Will in Voluntary Action" (1985). He recorded the exact time at which subjects consciously made the decision to move a finger at a moment of their choosing. An electroencephalogram monitoring brain activity revealed unconscious activity, which Libet called "readiness potential," an average of one half-second *before* participants were aware of their decision to move. In other words, before a person is aware of deciding to act, preparation for the action has already been initiated in the brain. Because of its philosophical implications for free will, this experiment has been thoroughly debated and repeated over the years, but for our purposes I will accept Libet's findings at face value and interpret them using the two-mind hypothesis.

 This half-second delay is explained by the proposition that our 300,000-year-old *Homo sapiens* individual consciousness only becomes self-aware in the act of experiencing itself from the underlying platform of our six-million-year-old collective consciousness. The decision is made freely by the new mind but must await its conscious registration in the old mind before knowledge (awareness) of the conscious decision is attained and reported.

The difficulty here for us moderns is that, when awareness is peeled off from consciousness, what's left is the naked reality of our individual intentions imprisoned within the fleeting instant of our feeling-consciousness. Then this difficulty is compounded because the old mind is also inaccessible (if not mentally ill) because it is the "background noise" of collective intentionality, within which we are immersed like fish unaware of the water in which we swim. As individuals our intimate engagement within this ubiquitous old mind experience is only apparent to us in the act of becoming aware of our private thoughts and motivations. We watch ourselves as individuals from the ancient intentions of our collective consciousness.

Animals are conscious of their felt experience as individuals but only our beloved dogs have the capacity to *share* their experience, because we bred them to do so. Pre modern hominins were only conscious of shared, collective experience because individual impulses of dominance and submission (ape mind) were all but entirely suppressed in the Freudian manner. Our two human minds are required for self-consciousness because it is produced by our *us* being conscious of our *me*. Albert Schweitzer wrote that, "True philosophy must start from the most immediate and comprehensive fact of consciousness: I am life that wants to live, in the midst of life that wants to live." (1949)

Mental illness: The price of awareness

I have opined at length on the function of anxiety among apes, who, like humans, also become depressed. Dr. Christiaan Barnard, the South African surgeon who performed the first heart transplant, told a story of two laboratory chimpanzees who lived in adjacent cages for several years. Dr. Barnard would often walk by them in the course of his busy day, vaguely noticing their playful antics. He did not give much thought to the resulting clamor when, one day, he and an assistant took away one of the animals to be "sacrificed" for experimental heart surgery. Some time later, as he walked by the remaining chimpanzee in his cage, he noticed it sitting motionless in the corner, obviously depressed. Dr. Barnard never again sacrificed a chimpanzee. He was deeply moved because he could empathize with the animal's existential response to separation in that he could feel it himself—he knows it well.

Much has been written about the sometimes-crippling anxiety conditions of dogs, mainly problems with separation and obsessive-compulsive disorder. Clearly, along with acquiring some of our cognitive abilities, they contracted some of our anxiety disorders. However, it is assumed that anxiety and depression in wild animals serve some adaptive function; if not, under the predominance of natural selection at the individual level, such ailments would long since have been swept away. When I first became interested in the relevance of evolution to psychiatry, I rejected outright the idea that major mental illnesses confer any benefits upon those who suffered from them, due to the magnitude of the disability they exact. I finally concluded that mental illnesses are an unavoidable epiphenomenon, a side effect of the unique features of human evolution.

Patients with panic disorder have told me, "I begin to feel anxious, and then I feel more anxious about being anxious," a process that rapidly ricochets with increasing intensity into panic. Once again, panic disorder is the pathological oscillation between the fear of separation and the fear of entrapment. Normally, these two fears regulate in tandem one's personal and social bonding. However, as these existential fears increase past a point of no return, the alarming experience of rapidly becoming *aware* of one's fears of separation and entrapment ratchets up their intensity until the patient becomes locked into frantically escaping from entrapment into separation and from separation into entrapment vibrating back and forth.[31]

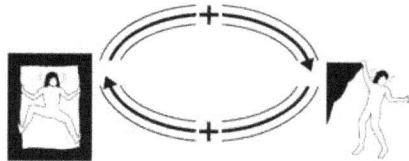

Normally *processing* such private emotions through experiencing them from a collective perspective is beneficial in many ways and is an essential dimension of psychoanalytic treatment. For many reasons, this conversion to awareness may not fully function, resulting in a buildup of these two unprocessed fears, but once they do start "coming out" into hyper-awareness under stress, both fears may devolve into feedback reverberation. Far from providing perspective and a healthy distance, escalating awareness now spins these two fears into an intolerable pitch, such that each fear frantically seeks solace by escaping into the other, back and forth. Mental illness opens a spigot of emotional awareness and hoses the deluge

---

[31] The fear of entrapment is claustrophobia, and the fear of separation is agoraphobia. Agoraphobia literally means "fear of the marketplace" and is translated as "fear of open spaces." However, my work with these patients convinced me that their root fear is separation.

back down the patient's throat. Awareness of our private feeling has conferred magical powers upon us, but it comes with the tragic price of mental illness.

Recall that risks of increased back and lower limb injury were worth the benefits of upright posture that made possible the revolutionary communication system that functions as the group's nervous system. Natural selection has reconstructed our back and lower limbs to the degree that our upright posture is pushing the envelope of what is possible to fashion from our knuckle-walking ape ancestors. Most do fine, but at the margins there is an irreducible price of back, hip, and knee problems that some must pay for our distinguished carriage.

In this same manner, nature has pushed the envelope of evolving regulatory mechanisms to maintain a dynamic balance in the interactions both within and between our two motivational mind systems. Accordingly, psychiatric disorders are the price extracted from our species for the miraculous benefits that the collaboration between two minds has bestowed upon us. This new functional paradigm could open new approaches to treatment.[32]

Prior to the evolution of *Homo sapiens*, no such regulation was necessary because everyone existed inside a shared communal mind that emanated from the authority of their groups. The old mind motivates through aversion, specifically to the fears of interpersonal separation, entrapment in the bottom/periphery of society, or the shame of banishment. In the old mind, the active agent is the group and its acted-upon object is the individual. By contrast, the new mind motivates the individual to seek pleasure produced by influencing the surrounding social world to respond. As the passion for vanity emerged in modern human individuals, the social anxieties that had always aversively motivated the communal mind evolved into a balance with the pleasure produced by individual self-esteem.

---

[32] The approach to the genetics of mental illness is altered by the possibility that these illnesses are functional disorders. The genes associated with these conditions are no longer viewed as pathological mutations, but as revealing scattered endemic short-comings in the regulation of an emotional system constantly pushed to its limits by the complexity and intensity of interaction between two minds, each comprised of very different agent-object/collective-individual dynamisms. Identifying a (hopefully) limited number of pathogenic permutations of otherwise normal genes could pro-duce maps of genetic vulnerability to a given mental illness.

Now, to cast this balance into a modern perspective, emotions generated by the new mind provide the excitement and romance of being human: enjoying our love lives, having and spending money, pursuing a hobby or artistic passion, the pursuit of recognition, success and happiness—the American Dream. But this fun side of our thoroughly modern lives is in balance with life's more serious aspects, circumscribed by anxieties at the prospect of poverty, the consequences of breaking the law, and the need to belong.

In health, mental process consists of a dynamic balance between being oriented by beliefs and values from the perspective of our groups and seeking the personal pleasure of the social approbation naturally arising from this integrated way of living. The emotionally serious tone of group authority and the beckoning music of our self-esteem mutually regulate one another. Besides this polarity in emotional quality, it is important to note the opposite *direction* of emotion and motivation in each of these interacting minds. The direction of a motivation is determined by the origin of its intentional source in relation to what it is "about." The group-mind is constantly orienting itself by receiving the continuous input of values and information from our nested groups outside us. To the degree that the group-mind influences our behavior, we act as the instruments and extensions of the intentions of our groups. By contrast, the motivations generated in the ego-mind flow directly out as the agency of behavior aimed at favorably influencing its object, which is our (mostly imagined) social audience. An emotional balance is maintained between these two very different motivations, one entering from our social environment and one exiting from the individual.

Melancholic depression is an example of an illness caused by an imbalance resulting from the failure of the new mind to regulate the old mind. As opposed to being motivated by self-display, a perfectly healthy, and indeed a culturally venerated form of ambition is when a person seeks to make more money than he needs due to the fear of falling back into poverty experienced as a youth. But then the esteem attained by having money alleviates and regulates that still underlying fear. In health, this balance between fear over the prospect of poverty and esteem from success can withstand inevitable financial ups and downs.

But if this individual is vulnerable to melancholia, perhaps due to a high level of anxiety regulated by esteem, the balance might be upset. An unexpected financial reversal can suddenly dip self-esteem below a threshold. Once the dike is breached, the patient is sucked into a pathologically intensified old mind dynamic between obedience and authority. The feelings of esteem that had flowed from the new mind's audience now turn to old mind persecution: the threat of banishment, and the public shame of poverty—the acute awareness of it—is felt to pour in on oneself from others.

In this feedback reverberation, the new mind is ensnared into pathologically intense awareness of the fear of being trapped in, and condemned to, poverty, which implodes in upon itself, crystallizing into a fixed delusion (false belief). In melancholia, fears that had been cushioned by esteem within the ego-mind devolve into the feedback reverberation of the old mind. From within the single-minded belief that banishment and humiliation are fitting comes the sense that "life is over." All boosters in the new mind have turned into old mind persecutors.

Mania is a failure of the old mind to regulate the new mind. Instead of a reversal, a sudden stroke of good fortune might trigger a manic episode. The flowing out of mental behavior motivated by attaining the euphoria of being intensely admired by others becomes so predominant that the new mind usurps the old mind. In the imbalance of this new mind pathology, the ego becomes inflated by co-opting the authority of the old mind, producing the experience of grandiosity that marshals the machinery of language, all aimed at an imagined swelling audience experienced as enraptured. Self-awareness disappears in mania. It is not difficult to empathize with mania because it is so thoroughly (modern) human. All of us have felt a touch of it when intoxicated by love or liquid spirits.

The two-mind perspective also lends insight into the enigmatic scourge of schizophrenia. As in the case of melancholia, in schizophrenia the old mind escapes regulation by the new mind. The extreme intensity of the normally unconscious dictates of authority in the old mind overwhelms and co-opts the ego-mind. Common to all schizophrenic thought is that the intentional direction of the self-conscious ego in relation to its imagined audience is reversed. Now the ego's formerly indistinct and passively benign "audience" whose function is to reflect esteem, is commandeered actively sending vividly distorted messages in the fragmented old mind's thought-language of belief—all specifically aimed squarely back at the individual. Like melancholia, schizophrenia is a pathological state of hyper-awareness.

As noted, the sources of incoming thoughts in schizophrenia range from commanding and authoritative old mind figures, such as God or government institutions, which are more likely to be experienced aversively, to new mind figures, such as pop stars or anonymous individuals typical of a normal ego's audience, all of whom are likely experienced as more benign, occasionally even amusing. Indeed, schizophrenic thoughts can actively flatter the patient's ego.

Perhaps the intransigence and chronicity of schizophrenia is the result of the sheer magnitude of old mind as compared to new mind. The old mind, although unconscious due to our collective immersion within it, is far more maturely developed and predominant than the newly appended ego-mind. In mania, when the young little fish swallows the old big fish, it becomes exhausted in time, coughs it back out, then collapses into protracted depression. Manic episodes are usually limited to about three to six months. However, when the big fish swallows the little fish in schizophrenia, it can digest it, and the old mind retains the capacity to function, soul to soul, in interpersonal relationships. But all too often, these relationships are managed in parallel with the ongoing experience of being bombarded by disordered thoughts from the forever-altered new mind audience. In schizophrenia, the old mind chronically usurps the patient's ego.

Stigma

While this essay introduces an understanding of human evolution through the lens of mental illness, its mission is to counter stigma. I have diagnosed the stigma of mental illness to be the result of contagion-fear triggered by our keen empathetic sensibilities' deep resonance with the symptoms. I have enlisted empathy as an instrument to discern that the inner experience of mental illnesses intimately connects us to the inner experience of our common ancestors. The same symptoms that cause the stigma of mental illness are vividly portrayed dimensions of the social environments that have been the felt collective soul of being human down through the ages.

So henceforth when you encounter major depression, you can regard that individual to be suffering from the power that transformed the law of the jungle into the law of right and wrong; and consider those who live with schizophrenia to be in the thrall of the collective consciousness within which we ascended from the animal kingdom into a "spiritual kingdom." Consider those in the grip of mania to be seized by the passionate desires that sling us headlong into a future, full of faith that the destiny of our six-million-year-old tribe will continue to stay on track.

Epilogue

The essay's portrait of human nature is not complete without this passage by Robert Bellah from his *Religion in Human Evolution* (2011) in which he exemplifies a causal relationship between collective instincts for justice and monotheistic religion. Bellah compares the trajectory of Zeus in Greece and that of Yahweh in Israel:

> As a thought experiment, in what might have been we can think of the close connection of Zeus and justice (dikē) beginning, tentatively, in Homer, becoming quite explicit in and central in Hesiod, powerfully applied to his immediate situation by Solon, and reiterated once again in the tragedies of Aeschylus. But although the concern for justice remains central for those we call the Presocratics, the connection with Zeus loosens drastically. We saw in the case of Israel that Yahweh emerged gradually from being one of many other gods, even the greatest god, to the status of the one and only true God. Zeus never underwent that fate, even though the possibility was never entirely lost: witness the *Hymn to Zeus* of the early third century BCE Stoic Cleanthes (p. 373).

Last three stanzas from Cleanthes' *Hymn to Zeus* (translated by E. H. Blakeney):

> O Thou most bounteous God that sittest throned
> In clouds, the Lord of lightning, save mankind
> From grievous ignorance!
> Oh, scatter it
> Far from their souls, and grant them to achieve
> True knowledge, on whose might Thou dost rely
> To govern all the world in righteousness;
>
> That so, being honoured, we may Thee requite
> With honour, chanting without pause Thy deeds,
> As all men should: since greater guerdon ne'er
> Befalls or man or god than evermore
> Duly to praise the Universal Law.

Acknowledgements

I am blessed to have Richard Gilbert as a brother-in-law. A writer, seeker, and fellow traveler, he has been with me every step of the way: from pondering my condensed "thought-pieces" in the early days to lovingly and passionately weighing in on all subsequent issues large and small. Richard, I cannot thank you enough.

The seasoned judgement, acute intelligence, and unfailing support of my remarkable wife Ann permeate this book.

My longtime colleague Patrick Lorenz initiated this essay when he suggested that I extract the ideas from my memoir into another book.

Patricia Lenihan skillfully edited the essay while adroitly tempering some of my untoward sensibilities.

I am deeply indebted to my old friend Jeffrey Weisberg for supporting my decision to embark on this journey some forty-five years ago.

I also appreciate design help from Martin Padley and my daughter Eva, copyediting from Eleanor Southworth, and many helpful suggestions from Mark Gall.

Read related essay by the author, "A Liberal Theory of Human Nature":

www.themontrealreview.com/2009/A-Liberal-Theory-Of-Human-Nature.php

Questions and comments welcome through "contact" on:

www.whywebecamehuman.com

Bibliography

Azuma H et al. (2007) "Postictal Suppression Correlates with Therapeutic Efficacy for Depression in Bilateral Sine and Pulse Wave ECT" *Psychiatry and Clinical Neurosciences* 61:168–173 [32][33]

Bauer SM et al. (2011) "Culture and the prevalence of hallucinations in schizophrenia" *Comprehensive Psychiatry*: 52(3): 319–325 [62]

Beck AT (1967) *The diagnosis and management of depression* Philadelphia: U of Pennsylvania Press [21]

Bekoff M, Pierce J (2009) *Wild Justice: The Moral Lives of Animals* Chicago: U of Chicago Press [88]

Bellah RN (2011) *Religion in Human Evolution: From the Paleolithic to the Axial Age* Cambridge, Harvard U Press [131]

Berger L (2017) *Almost Human: The Astonishing Tale of Homo naledi and the Discovery That Changed Our Human Story* Washington: National Geographic [96]

Bleuler E (1950) *Dementia Praecox or the Group of Schizophrenias* New York, International U Press [60-62]

Boaz NT, Ciochon RL (2004) *Dragon Bone Hill, An Ice-Age Saga of Homo Erectus* New York: Oxford U Press [69]

Boehm C (2012) *Moral Origins, The Evolution of Virtue, Altruism, and Shame* New York: Basic Books [91]

Bonanni A et al. (2010) "Effect of Affiliative and Agonistic Relationships on Leadership Behavior in Free-Ranging Dogs" *Animal Behavior* 79 no. 5: 981–991 [96]

Bowles S (2009) "Did Warfare Among Ancestral Hunter Gatherers Affect the Evolution of Human Social Behaviors?" *Science* 324: 1293-1298 [65]

Brainstorm Consortium (2018) "Analysis of shared heritability in common disorders of the brain" *Science* 360 Issue 6395 [12]

Bramble DM, Leiberman, D E (2004) "Endurance running and the evolution of Homo" *Nature* 432: 345–352 [87]

Brown JM, Atardi LD (2005) "The role of apoptosis in cancer development and treatment response" *Nature Reviews Cancer* 5: 231–237 [33]

Buber M (1958) *I and Thou* New York: Scribner [124]

Byrne RW, Whitten A (1988) *Machiavellian Intelligence* Oxford, Oxford U Press [73]

Chakravarti A (2010) "Genomics is not enough" *Science* 334:15 [13]

Cheney DL, Seyfarth RM (2007) *Baboon Metaphysics: The Evolution of a Social Mind* Chicago: U of Chicago Press [79]

Crivelli C et al. (2016) "Reading Emotions from Faces in Two Indigenous Societies," Journal of Experimental Psychology: General 145, no. 7: 830–43 [6]

---

[33] Page references to this book are in brackets at end of each citation

Damasio A (1999) *The Feeling of What Happens: Body and Emotion in the Making of Consciousness* Orlando: Harcourt [120]

Darwin C (1859) *On the Origin of Species by Means of Natural Selection* New York: London: John Murray [119]

Darwin C (1860) Letter to Asa Gray *Darwin Correspondence Project* (#2743) Cambridge UK [84]

Darwin C (1871) *The Descent of Man and Selection in Relation to Sex* New York: London: John Murray [84, 86, 109, 123]

Darwin C (1872) *The Expression of the Emotions in Man and Animals* London: John Murray [5]

Dawkins R (1976) *The Selfish Gene* Oxford: Oxford U Press [68, 70]

De Becker G (1997) *The Gift of Fear: Survival Signals that Protect Us from Violence* New York: Dell [54]

De Waal F (1982) *Chimpanzee Politics* Baltimore: Johns Hopkins U Press [52]

Delay JP, Deniker P, Harl JM (1952) "Therapeutic use in psychiatry of phenothiazine of central elective action" *Ann Med Psychol* (Paris) 110(21):112–117 [56]

Díaz-Muñoz SL, Bales K (2013) "'Monogamy' in Primates: Variability, Trends and Synthesis" *Am J Primatology* 78(3): 283-287 [83]

Dugatkin LA, Trut L (2017) *How to Tame a Fox (and Build a Dog): Visionary Scientists and a Siberian Tale of Jump-Started Evolution* Chicago: U of Chicago Press [109]

Dunbar RIM (1992) "Neocortex size as a constraint on group size in primates" *Journal of Human Evolution* 20:469-493 [99,100]

Dunbar RIM, Shultz, S (2007) "Evolution in the Social Brain" *Science* 317:1344–1347 [100]

Ekman P (2007) *Emotions Revealed, Second Edition: Recognizing Faces and Feelings to Improve Communication and Emotional Life* New York, Holt [6]

Ekman P (2013) *Emotion in the Human Face* Cambridge, MA: Malor Books [6]

Eldredge N, Gould SJ (1972) "Punctuated equilibria: An alternative to phyletic gradualism" *Models in paleobiology* Edited by Schopf TJM. San Francisco: Freeman, Cooper, 82–115. [79]

Ferenczi EM et al. (2016) "Prefrontal cortical regulation of brainwide circuit dynamics and reward-related behavior" *Science* 351 no. 6268 [28]

Fisher RA (1930) *The Genetical Theory of Natural Selection* New York: Dover [85]

Fitch WT (2010) *The Evolution of Language* Cambridge: Cambridge University Press [109, 122]

Gavrilets S (2012) "Human origins and the transition from promiscuity to pair-bonding" *Proceedings of the National Academy of Sciences* 109:9923–9928 [83]

Gibbons A (2014) "How we tamed ourselves—and became modern" *Science* 346:405-406 [110]

Gorman J et al. (1984) "Response to Hyperventilation in a Group of Patients with Panic Disorder" *American Journal of Psychiatry* 141(7):857–861 [48]

Grice HP (1975) "Logic and Conversation" In *The Logic of Grammar,* edited by Davidson D, Harman G. Encino, CA: Dickenson, 65 [122]

Haidt J (2012) *The Righteous Mind: Why Good People Are Divided by Politics and Religion* New York, Pantheon [63]

Hamilton MJ et al. (2009) "Population stability, cooperation, and the invasibility of the human species" *PNAS* 106 no. 30: 12255–12260 [98]

Hamilton W (1964) "The genetical evolution of social behaviour I and II" *Journal of Theoretical Biology* 7 (1): 1–52 [68]

Hauser MD, Chomsky N, Fitch WT (2002) "The Faculty of Language: What Is It, Who Has It, and How Did It Evolve?" *Science* 298:1569–1579 [123]

Hilker R, et al. (2018) "Heritability of Schizophrenia and Schizophrenia Spectrum Based on the Nationwide Danish Twin Register" *Biological Psychiatry* 83: 492-498 [12]

Hrdy SB (2006) *Evolutionary context of human development: The cooperative breeding model. In Attachment and Bonding: A New Synthesis*, ed. Carter CS, Ahnert I, Grossmann KE, Hrdy SB, Lamb ME, Porges SW, and Sachser N, Cambridge, MA: MIT Press: 9-32 [89]

Hublin JJ, et al. (2017) "New fossils from Jebel Irhoud, Morocco and the pan-African origin of *Homo sapiens*" *Nature* 546: 289-292, Extended Data Figure 5: "Facial and endocranial shape differences among Homo groups" [110]

Hughes WOH, Oldroyd BP, Beekman M, Ratneiks LW (2008) "Ancestral Monogamy Shows Kin Selection Is Key to the Evolution of Eusociality" *Science* (320):1213–1216 [82]

Jackendoff R (2002) *Foundations of Language: Brain, Meaning, Grammar, Evolution* New York: Oxford U Press, 427 [108]

Jung CG (1961) *Freud and Psychoanalysis* Bollingen Series XX. Princeton: Princeton U Press, 339 [93]

Kallmann, F (1946) "The Genetic Theory of Schizophrenia: An analysis of 691 twin index families" *American Journal of Psychiatry* 103: 309-322 [11, 12]

Kaminski J et al. (2008) "Domestic Dogs Are Sensitive to a Human's Perspective." *Behavior* 146:979–998 [121]

Keeley LH (1996) *War Before Civilization: The Myth of the Peaceful Savage* New York: Oxford U Press [64]

Klein D (1993) "False Suffocation Alarms, Spontaneous Panics, and Related Conditions: An Integrated Approach" *Archives of General Psychiatry* 50(4):306–317 [23, 48]

Laland KN (2017) *Darwin's Unfinished Symphony: How Culture Made the Human Mind* Princeton: Princeton U Press [113]

Libet B (1985) "Unconscious Cerebral Initiative and the Role of Conscious Will in Voluntary Action" *Behavioral and Brain Sciences* 8:529–566 [120]

Lovejoy CO (1981) "The Origin of Man" *Science* 111:341–350 [83]

Lovejoy CO (2009) "Reexamining Human Origins in Light of *Ardipithecus ramidus*" *Science* 26: 74e1–78 [83]

Mayberg HS et al. (2005) "Deep Brain Stimulation for Treatment-Resistant Depression" *Neuron* 45: 651–660 [32]

McCrae RR, John OP (1992) "An introduction to the five-factor model and its applications" *Journal of Personality* 60: 175 [12]

Mendel G (1866) "Versuche über Pfanzenhybriden." *Verhandlungen naturforschenden Vereins Brünn* 4 [28]

Miller G (2000) *The Mating Mind: How Sexual Choice Shaped the Evolution of Human Nature.* New York: Doubleday [106]

Miller G (2012) "Why Is Mental Illness So Hard to Treat?" *Science* 338: 32-33 [11]

Nasar S (1998) *A Beautiful Mind: The Life of Mathematical Genius and Nobel Laureate John Nash* New York: Simon & Schuster p. 260 [108]

Nesse R (2019) *Good Reasons for Bad Feelings: Insights from the Frontier of Evolutionary Psychiatry* New York: Penguin. [5]

Nesse R (1990) "The evolutionary functions of repression and the go defenses" *Journal of the American Academy of Psychoanalysis* 18(2): 260-285 [5]

Northoff G (2009) "Differential parametric modulation of self-relatedness and emotions in different brain regions" *Human Brain Mapping* 30:369–382 [32]

Olivieri A et al. (2006) "The mtDNA Legacy of the Levantine Early Upper Paleolithic in Africa" *Science* 314:1767–1770 [98]

Okhovat M, Berrio A, Wallace G, Ophir AG, Phelps M (2015) "Sexual fidelity trade-offs promote regulatory variation in the prairie vole brain" *Science* 350:1371–1374 [82]

Opie C, Atkinson QD, Shultz S (2012) "The evolutionary history of primate mating systems" *Communicative & Integrative Biology* 5:458–461 [83]

Pitts M, Roberts M (1998) *Fairweather Eden: Life half a million years ago as revealed by the excavations at Boxgrove* New York: Fromm Internat'l [98]

Prado-Martinez J et al. (2013) "Great ape genetic diversity and population history" *Nature* 499: 471–475 [81]

Prüfer K et al. (2014) "The complete genome sequence of a Neanderthal from the Altai Mountains" *Nature* 505: 43–49 [114]

Prum RO (2017) *The Evolution of Beauty: How Darwin's Forgotten Theory of Mate Choice Shapes the Animal World - and Us* New York: Doubleday [110]

Rabins P (2013) *The Why of Things: Causality in Science, Medicine, and Life* New York: Columbia U Press [4]

Range F, Virányi Z (2014) "Tracking the evolutionary origins of dog-human cooperation: the 'Canine Cooperation Hypothesis'" *Frontiers of Psychology* 5: 1582 [96]

Ryle G (1949) *The Concept of Mind* London: Hutchinson's University Library [116]

Sakin HA (1999) "The Anticonvulsant Hypothesis of the Mechanisms of Action of ECT: Current Status" *Journal of ECT* 15: 5–26 [31]

Sacks, O (2017) *The River of Consciousness* New York: Knoff [112]

Seyfarth RM, Cheney DL (2003) "Signalers and Receivers in Animal Communication" *Annual Review of Psychology* 54: 145–173 [117]

Sapolsky RM (2017) *Behave: The Biology of Humans at Our Best and Worst* New York: Penguin Press [100]

Schweitzer A (1949) *The Philosophy of Civilization* New York: MacMillan [121]

Seeley TD (2010) *Honeybee Democracy* Princeton: Princeton U Press [105]

Shultz S, Opie C, Atkinson QD (2011) "Stepwise evolution of stable sociality" *Nature* 479: 219–224 [110]

Sikora M, et al. (2017) "Ancient genomes show social and reproductive behavior of early Upper Paleolithic foragers" *Science* 358: 659-662 [114]

Silk J (2007) "Social Components of Fitness in Primate Groups" *Science* 317: 1347–1351 [89]

Smith A (1776) *The Wealth of Nations* London: W. Strahan and T. Cadell [88]

Smith A (1759) *The Theory of Moral Sentiments* Edinburgh: Alexander Kincaid and J. Bell [88]

Smith M, Szathmáry E (1995) *The Major Transitions in Evolution* Oxford: Oxford U Press [93]

Smith WC (1977) *Belief and History* Charlottesville: UVA Press [64]

Smutts BB, Gubernick DJ (1992) "Male-Infant Relationships in Nonhuman Primates: Paternal Investment or Mating Effort" In *Father-Child Relationships: Cultural and Biosocial Contexts.* Edited by Hewlett BS. New York: Walter de Gruyter [83]

Solomon A (2001) *The Noonday Demon: An Atlas of Depression* New York: Scribner [30, 61]

Solomon A (2012) *Far from the Tree: Parents, Children, and the Search for Identity* New York: Scribner [64]

Strandburg-Peshkin A, Farine DR, Couzin ID, Margaret C. Crofoot (2015) "Shared decision-making drives collective movement in wild baboons" *Science* 348: 1358–1361 [95]

Styron W (1990) *Darkness Visible: A Memoir of Madness* New York: Random House [38]

Thompson WM (1859) *The Land and the Book* London: T Nelson and Sons [2]

Tomasello M (1999) *The Cultural Origins of Human Cognition* Cambridge, MA: Harvard U Press [121]

Tomasello M (2014) *A Natural History of Human Thinking* Cambridge, MA: Harvard U Press, 153 [1, 2]

Tomasello M (2019) *Becoming Human: A Theory of Ontogeny* Cambridge: Harvard U Press [91-93]

Torrey EF, Yolken RH (2010) "Psychiatric Genocide: Nazi Attempts to Eradicate Schizophrenia" *Schizophrenia Bulletin* 36: 26-32 [11]

Trivers R L (1971) "The Evolution of Reciprocal Altruism" *The Quarterly Review of Biology* 46 (1): 35–57 [68]

Ungar PS (2017) *Evolution's Bite: A Story of Teeth, Diet, and Human Origins* Princeton: Princeton U Press [97]

Weiss A, et al (2011) "Overview of Emergency Department Visits in the United States, 2011" Healthcare Cost and Utilization Project, Statistical Brief #174. [94]

Wilson DS, Wilson EO (2007) "Rethinking the Theoretical Foundation of Sociobiology" *Quarterly Review of Biology*, 82(4):327–348 [66-69]

Wilson EO (2012) *The Social Conquest of Earth* New York: W. W. Norton [69]

Wittgenstein L (1953) *Philosophical Investigations* Malden, MA: Blackwell [122]

Wylie, JV (2010) *Diagnosing and Treating Mental Illness: A Guide for Physicians, Nurses, Patients, and Their Families* Spokane: Demers Books. Second edition (2012) [26]

www.ingramcontent.com/pod-product-compliance
Lightning Source LLC
Chambersburg PA
CBHW081647270326
41933CB00018B/3376